Journeys in Healing

How others have triumphed over
disease and disability

Dr Shaun Matthews

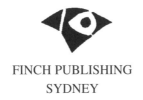

FINCH PUBLISHING
SYDNEY

> *To my father,*
> *Michael Matthews,*
> *who taught me the*
> *importance of listening*

Journeys in Healing

This edition first published in 2003 in Australia and New Zealand by Finch Publishing Pty Limited, PO Box 120, Lane Cove, NSW 1595, Australia.
ABN 49 057 285 248

05 04 03   8 7 6 5 4 3 2 1

Copyright © 2003 Shaun Matthews

The author asserts his moral rights in this work throughout the world without waiver. All rights reserved. No part of this publication may be reproduced, stored in a retrieval system or transmitted in any form or by any means (electronic or mechanical, through reprography, digital transmission, recording or otherwise) without the prior written permission of the publisher.

National Library of Australia Cataloguing-in-Publication entry

> Matthews, Shaun.
> Journeys in healing: how others have triumphed over
> disease and disability.
> Bibliography.
> Includes index.
> ISBN 1 876451 42 4.
> 1. Sick – Biography. 2. Sick – Psychology. 3. Healing. I.
> Title.
> 362.10922

Edited by Marie-Louise Taylor
Editorial assistance from Sheila Mayer
Text designed and typeset in Giovanni 10/14.
Internal design by Warren Ventures
Cover design by saso content and design
Cover photograph courtesy of gettyimages
Illustrations by Susan Boyle
Printed by BPA Print Group

Disclaimer While every care has been taken in researching and compiling the information in this book, it is in no way intended to replace consultation with a qualified health care professional. Readers are encouraged to seek such help as they deem necessary. The author and publisher specifically disclaim any liability arising from the application of information in this book.

Other Finch titles can be viewed at **www.finch.com.au**

Contents

Foreword by Dr Ian Gawler   *v*

Introduction   *1*

Part I   **The Interviews**

Nicki's story   14
'Close to death, you remember only the good times.'

Rebecca's story   30
'It was my saving grace that this thing came along to help me be not as I was.'

Anna's story   47
'The journey of healing, if it's a worthwhile and real healing, is a journey of learning.'

Peter's story   67
'What is important is how much healing has happened. And that may mean I don't get cured.'

Kathryn's story   83
'The very thing that probably causes the illness in the first place – that inner drive, that perfectionism – also encourages you to want to be well again.'

Janelle's story   104
'For healing to happen, you have to let go of whatever the story was about why you got sick.'

Sara's story   120
'I thought when I was lying in traction, "Okay, I'm not going to be able to run away from things any more."'

Shankardev's story   132
'In the process of the illness and suffering, a lot of insights can come.'

Part II	What we can learn	
	Getting proactive	148
	Living with serious illness	160
	The road to recovery	168
	Healing as learning	175
	Healing the whole person	185
	The gift of illness	195
Part III	A physician's own experience	
	Beyond medical school	202
	Physician heal thyself	218

Conclusion	237
Appendix: A story of ancient healing in the modern world	240
Glossary	243
Acknowledgements	246
Further reading	247
Index	249

Foreword

We live in changing times. Challenging times. Interesting times! It is not so long since doctors were regarded as gods. Their authority over illness was not questioned; their word was final. Currently the capacity of many doctors to even practise medicine is under threat because they are being sued so often and for so much.

In recent decades the nature of medicine has changed. A century ago, the doctor often filled the role of physician, teacher, confidant, even priest. More recently, medicine has become more fixated upon science, the workings of the body as a mechanical object, the role of drugs, and physical interventions like surgery.

Much of this has been good. People live longer, more diseases appear to be treatable, there is less quackery; but still it seems clear to most that something important is missing. What of the emotions, the mind and the spirit? What about the person who has the disease? What about the human story that places the disease in the midst of a dynamic, vibrant, sometimes chaotic, sometimes poetic, invariably moving landscape?

Shaun Matthews is one of the current wave of doctors establishing a new paradigm for medicine. In a way, this new approach is reverting to that older style of medicine, incorporating the compassion, the time to listen, the time to care, that we romantically remember of the old-style GPs doing their house calls.

But there is more. Science is being incorporated, integrated into the caring, human face of medicine to create a truly holistic approach.

And there is a clear new emphasis. Instead of directly telling the patient what to do, the new doctors are taking the time to listen. In listening, they hear remarkable stories.

Shaun has done a great service by not only listening to, but also recording the stories of some truly remarkable patients. Perhaps it is more politically correct to speak of 'people dealing with disease', as these patients provide insights, humour, pathos and inspiration as they share their incredible lives.

Shaun offers the book 'as a focus for reflection on the nature of healing'. The stories flow easily in conversational style. The questions with which Shaun prompts those interviewed could well provide a model for doctors interested in learning how to draw out a person's story. What they do for the reader is to lead into a wonderful exploration of how different people with different illnesses found their own unique ways to firstly cope, then to overcome and live with their condition.

'Healing is necessarily a highly individual process, and in simple terms, what works for some will often not work for others,' Shaun writes. But there are common themes. Some memorable quotes:

You can 'see your health issue as an opportunity or a curse. You can use your condition either to grow or to become totally self-absorbed and indulgent.'

'You've got to want to get better because it doesn't really matter what you do, if mentally you don't want to get well, you won't get well.'

And, '… the ultimate healing state is complete self-acceptance and self-love and, similarly, complete acceptance and love for others, for all beings.'

How people faced with major health challenges came to these views – the struggles they faced, then the moments of clarity and insight – forms the basis of this book.

I highly recommend *Journeys in Healing*. These human stories, prompted and drawn out by a caring, sensitive doctor, make compelling, inspiring and instructive reading. Read this book and feel your heart being warmed!

Dr Ian Gawler OAM
Executive Director, The Gawler Foundation
November 2002

Introduction

As a medical practitioner who has also trained in various forms of 'alternative' medicine, I have been privileged to meet with patients whose presence and example have affected me profoundly. To sit with them, to share in some of their insights and to feel a little of their pain has been a rich gift to me both personally and professionally. Their courage in the face of adversity arising in the context of serious illness has humbled me and their creative approaches opened my eyes to how much we have still to learn about the mysteries of healing. At the end of such consultations I often feel like a novice student awed by the wise words of a great and unexpected teacher.

My regret at such times is that more people are not able to draw sustenance, as I have done, from their experience. The impulse to put together a book such as this is largely derived from this sense of dissatisfaction. At a time in the history of medicine when the limitations of a materialist paradigm of health are being sorely questioned it seems timely that the experiencer of the disease finds a place to speak.

In essence this is a book based on experience: not the experience of highly qualified and learned doctors in clinical practice, nor the statistical experience resulting from controlled clinical trials; but the experience of ordinary people who have responded to the challenge of potentially life-threatening or debilitating illnesses in remarkable ways. These individuals have demonstrated extraordinary capacities for healing and have been courageous enough to share their stories with the general public.

On another level this book explores the very human side of healing, so often not talked about because of shame and embarrassment. The feelings of helplessness and dependency, the lurking fear that one may never again function normally and the lack of self-esteem that comes with chronic illness are issues rarely touched on in the doctor–patient relationship. The isolation that results from not wanting to be perceived as a whinger and yet having pressing physical and/or emotional needs is another experience not easily grasped by even the best intentioned of caregivers. As such, the candid and very personal accounts of those interviewed highlight some important aspects of what it means to be chronically ill.

Since leaving the hospital system eight years ago I have been determined to continue my education in healing through a study of 'alternative' medicine. Disillusioned with the modern view of health, which largely focuses on the physical aspects of disease, I delved into an approach to healing that encompasses the many dimensions of what it is to be human. In attempting to address this deficiency in my understanding my search has taken me into body-oriented psychotherapy, different forms of massage, meditation, iridology, diet, Ayurveda, the traditional medicine of India, and yoga.

My medical practice is particularly oriented towards people suffering from chronic illnesses who are interested in contributing to their own recovery. My approach to encouraging healing is thus a blend of all these different systems. A consultation could therefore involve: an in-depth review of a patient's diet; instruction in some yoga poses to promote the flow of energy around the body; the prescription of some herbs to nourish depleted tissues in the body; the making of an audiotape encouraging deep relaxation; or sometimes the exploration of a deeply held belief system that is impeding that person's development as a human being. In this context I have come to appreciate the inherently complementary nature of these approaches to healing and find the term 'complementary medicine' a more apt way of describing those approaches not currently part of mainstream medical practice.

The word 'holistic' in the description of medical and health care practice also deserves some mention at this point. Holistic, as I understand it, signifies an approach to the person coming for treatment that is inclusive of the many dimensions of what it means to be a human being. In practical terms it is an approach that takes into consideration the physical, emotional, mental and spiritual levels of human existence. Importantly, it acknowledges the profound interconnections between these different levels and how they fundamentally influence each other.

In my experience, however, there are many health care practitioners, both mainstream and complementary, who claim to be holistic in orientation but whose approach is a lot less comprehensive in its application. How often do we hear of acupuncturists who stick needles in their patients, prescribe herbs and send the patient on their way; naturopaths who prescribe a host of vitamins and herbs but know very little about the interior world of their client; or medical practitioners whose idea of holistic health care is to include a dietary and lifestyle assessment in addition to their medical consultation?

In the chapter entitled 'Healing the whole person' the subject of holistic approaches to health is explored in more detail, drawing from the experience of the individuals interviewed in the book.

Experience is the best teacher

The compiling and writing of this book took on a personal relevance for me when, after twelve years in medical practice, I found myself facing many of the same issues as my patients. Two years of unusual abdominal pain, having been variously diagnosed as irritable bowel syndrome, Crohn's disease and a gall bladder condition, was eventually discovered to be three amoebic ulcers of my large bowel, most likely a legacy of my sojourns in India when working and studying there in the previous decade. The anxiety of not knowing what was wrong was brought home to me in a very real way; a way that I could not possibly have foreseen. In the final chapter of this book, entitled 'Physician heal thyself', I include my own experiences of having a serious chronic illness and some personal insights into healing.

Coming face to face with the diagnosis of a serious disease is a profound experience. The dimensions of that experience and what it means to that person can never really be known by anyone else. There is necessarily a separation created between the person with the diagnosis and their most intimate friends, family members and the most compassionate of health care practitioners. For people in this situation the sympathetic ear of a caregiver, whether professional or lay, can never replace the sense of connection that can sometimes arise when in the company of someone with a similar condition. Those who have participated in support groups for people with chronic illness or in twelve-step programs can testify to this.

Many of us will have been confronted at some time with the impossible-to-answer questions of children. Their minds fresh and untainted by convention, they have a marvellous capacity to ask the unimaginable: 'Mum, what does a strawberry taste like?' At this point, assuming there are no strawberries in the house, we may resort to comparisons with the taste of other fruit. Alternatively, we could give a description of the taste of a strawberry: 'Well, it's sweet, moist and delicious.' However, it's difficult not to feel the inadequacy of one's attempts to convey to their inquiring minds something seemingly so simple. Even with the vocabulary and craft of Wordsworth, the most inspired description is likely to fall well short of actually giving the child a fresh, ripe strawberry. Such is the nature of experience.

Experience as the best teacher has long been recognised. The value of knowledge derived from experience was particularly prized by a group of Greek physicians. The Empirici, as they called themselves, lived in the third century BC and drew their rules of practice entirely from experience. At a time when philosophical speculation and irrelevant scientific experimentation was rife, direct experience was much valued. The English word 'empirical' comes to us from the Greek word *empeirikos*, meaning experienced.

In educational circles this point is now receiving more attention as different types of learning are being differentiated. Intellectually-based learning has held sway at schools and universities for hundreds of years. Certainly this style of learning comprised a large portion of my own education during six years of medical school. However, educationalists are increasingly coming to value experiential learning in the training of students. This point has always been well appreciated in the apprenticeship approach to learning where the acquisition of practical skills is critical to one's vocational development.

In my own case I well remember the adage touted by my superiors in hospital internship training: 'Watch one, do one, teach one.' This was dramatically reinforced on the second day of my medical career when I was taught how to insert an intercostal chest tube in the morning (to expel trapped air, a plastic tube is passed through the skin and the muscles between the ribs into the space created when a lung has collapsed). That afternoon I was required to perform the same procedure on an unconscious patient in the middle of a cardiac arrest.

Set amidst the incessant beeping of cardiac monitors, the flurry of nurses darting around the arrest trolley in search of syringes and injectable medicines and the gaze of five senior colleagues, my body was soon tense with anticipation. Then there was the realisation that one of the lungs of the man we were trying to resuscitate had collapsed. Next I heard the casualty director announce that Dr Matthews would now insert an intercostal catheter. For a split second I wondered who this Dr Matthews was before realising that my passive role in the proceedings had abruptly ended. With the sweat now pouring down my back I feverishly scrubbed up and ineptly struggled to get my rubber gloves on. Inserting the tube, sheathed around a metal trochar (not unlike a knitting needle), proved to be more difficult than I remembered and not helped by the taunts of some of my colleagues – 'Watch out for the heart!' Acutely self-conscious at having my clinical inexperience exposed before all and sundry, I remember feeling inadequate and a little humiliated. As it turned out I did successfully introduce the intercostal tube and drain off the trapped air in his chest, though despite our best efforts we were unable to bring the man back to life.

As a final year medical student struggling to keep abreast of the latest developments in medicine, I would regularly peruse the leading medical journals of the Western world. Only one article still sticks in my memory. It was in the form of a letter to the editor of the *British Medical Journal* from a physician who had spent six weeks in an Intensive Care Unit after suffering a blood clot to his lung. Despite having worked in a teaching hospital for twenty years and visiting Intensive Care on a regular basis, nothing had prepared him for the experience of being a patient in these circumstances. His thoughts and feelings, bearing the authenticity of personal experience, not surprisingly made a greater impression on me than all of the other articles I read that year.

For me his letter highlights the gap between knowledge and understanding based on direct personal experience and that derived from indirect experience and the intellect – a gap that separates sufferers of disease from their closest friends and caregivers. Can we do anything to reduce this gap? And if so, how? These are questions that need to be addressed in the education of health care practitioners and in the community as a whole.

In the field of drug and alcohol counselling it has been recognised for some time that the best counsellors are often people who have successfully learnt how to deal with their own addictions. In coming to terms with the addictive aspects of their personality and participating in their own recovery, they have much to offer others struggling with substance abuse. The inherent value of their hard-won personal experience is acknowledged and put to good use.

Many of these counsellors will have benefited from support group meetings, perhaps along the lines of the twelve-step program first established by Alcoholics Anonymous. The inherent value of being able to share one's innermost secrets in a safe and supportive environment and the sense of connection to other group members who have shared their experience is well recognised. It is unfortunate that there are not more opportunities for sufferers of chronic diseases to come together in this way; though I anticipate there will be significant developments in this area in the not too distant future.

Sadly, the art of medicine has become the poor cousin in an age dominated by medical technology and statistics. Medicine as a science is eagerly embraced by doctors today, who are often slow to give credence to the observations and opinions of their patients. In an age of increasing accessibility to information and patient education, such a narrow-minded attitude seems profoundly contrary to the growth of our knowledge and understanding of health and disease. Indeed, one of the distinguishing features of the approach of Hippocrates, the father of Western clinical medicine, was the profound reverence he gave to the claims of his patients.

It is readily apparent to doctors and the general public that the causes of many chronic diseases, including cancer and autoimmune diseases such as systemic lupus erythematosis (SLE) and rheumatoid arthritis, are still not well understood. Many of the survival rates for major cancers, including cancers of the lung, stomach and pancreas, have not changed appreciably in the past 30 years. In the case of lung cancer there is an 11–15 percent chance of being alive five years after diagnosis. The figures for cancer of the pancreas are even bleaker; the five-year survival rate is only 4–5 percent. Given the limitations of our present paradigm of health, it seems reasonable for members of the general public to look more widely for therapeutic options to incurable and chronic diseases.

Figures from the United States show that this is just what they are doing. In 1993 a landmark survey by the Harvard Medical School showed that one-third of Americans used non-traditional therapies. And, according to the National Center for Complementary and Alternative Medicine, by 1997, 42 per cent of US health care users spent US$27 billion a year on these therapies. The Australian experience is little different: a study in South Australia carried out in 1996 found that almost 50 per cent of Australians over 15 years of age had used at least one non-medically prescribed complementary medication annually.

In response to growing consumer demand for complementary medicine, a panel convened by the Office of Alternative Medicine at the National Institutes of Health in the US recommended that all medical and nursing students be exposed to alternative theories and techniques. At least fifty of the US's 135 medical schools are supplementing traditional subjects such as physiology and anatomy with acupuncture, homeopathy, massage, nutrition and prayer.

In this context it seems appropriate that a book devoted to individuals who have approached their own healing in innovative and creative ways should be made available. What follows are necessarily very personal and unique approaches to recovery based on first-hand experience. The individuals interviewed for this book came to my attention in a number of ways; some had been patients of mine, some were colleagues who came forward on hearing about the nature of the book I was writing, while others were recommended to me by friends who felt that the stories of the individuals concerned would help to enrich the book. Three of those interviewed were friends of mine whose healing through major illness had been the subject of many discussions over the years.

In approaching the task of editing the transcripts of the interviews, I have attempted to limit my editing as much as possible in order that the reader can get a feeling for the person being interviewed. Too often, in my experience, transcripts of interviews are 'cleaned up' in the editing process and one is left with a story that is missing some level of authenticity or may read as being a little too good to be true. So I have left in portions of text that might be deemed by some people to be irrelevant to the question of how best to facilitate healing. I hope that this 'warts and all' approach to editing will serve to emphasise the very human side of the people interviewed for this book.

Making room for the individual

One of the significant advances in the history of Western science was the pairing of mathematics and medicine. Using numbers to improve diagnostic and therapeutic efficacy was first used in France in the late eighteenth century. Using statistical analyses, physicians and surgeons were able to gauge the success of therapeutic interventions. This tradition has been further developed so that the survival figures of all kinds of life-threatening diseases are currently available to doctors. While such information can be useful in gauging the seriousness of the diagnosis, it often reinforces a very limited view as to what is possible in terms of recovery. Many people when faced with a medical statistic telling them there is a 90 percent chance they will be dead in five years time will effectively begin a psychological decline there and then.

I believe the psychic impact of such statistical prognoses cannot be overestimated in our present age. To the average person a powerful doctor quoting such a statistic is akin to having a death bone pointed in their direction. In this matter, my thinking has been influenced by Dr Ian Gawler who maintains that the prognosis must necessarily remain an unknown quantity. Much will depend on the individual's capacity to mobilise their own innate healing force, if long-term survival is desired.

Healing is a complex phenomenon. In spite of the tremendous advances in medical science in the twentieth century there are still many aspects of healing that we do not understand. Such is the nature of life and its mysteries. Certainly I see healing as more than just the recovery from physical disease. By focusing exclusively on the physical plane of existence we reduce the complexity of the human condition immeasurably.

This point was brought home to me in a very real way by one of my patients several years ago. Indeed my initial thought to assemble a book such as this was triggered by this same man. Phillip was referred to me by a medical colleague in 1994 for help with his meditation practice. He had been diagnosed the previous year with bowel cancer. Several months later further tests showed that he had developed secondary spread of the cancer to his lungs. He was told the cancer was inoperable. Unfortunately, chemotherapy had caused severe side effects and had been suspended for the time being. Despite all these setbacks Phillip was keen to improve his situation and interested in furthering his practice of meditation. At the time he was meeting with a Buddhist monk and taking steps to confront his own death.

I taught Phillip a series of meditations, some with a specific healing focus and others of a more general nature. Phillip was enthusiastic and practised them assiduously, as well as regularly attending the Buddhist meditation group. It was not long before I noticed a marked change in his demeanour; Phillip would arrive at our sessions with a palpable aura of contentment. He would tell me that having cancer had transformed his view of life in the most positive way.

He now was simply thankful for each day and was enjoying the time available to him. The change in Phillip's demeanour was also noted by his referring doctor with some amazement. But for me, what was most striking was Phillip's presence. During our sessions together I could not help but be moved by his gentle warmth and humility. He seemed to radiate a quality that is difficult to describe but impossible to mistake. In short, I felt that he had achieved tremendous internal peace in the midst of his terminal illness. Time had lost its grip on him.

Three months after beginning our work together, Phillip's cancer specialist ordered further chest X-rays, which showed no further growth in the lung secondary deposits. We were both pleased and as his healing practices were well established we agreed to meet again when necessary. As it turned out I did not see Phillip for another year and a half.

I mention Phillip's story for two reasons: because of the remission that was produced in the context of an intensive self-healing practice; and because much of his healing seemed to be taking place at the mental and spiritual levels of his being, physical survival having become a secondary concern to him for a time.

Structure of this book

Part I of this book is made up of transcripts of interviews with eight individuals who have chosen to take an active role in their own healing. All the interviews took place in the privacy of their own homes and all those interviewed were offered the right of editing anything in the transcripts they did not feel comfortable with having published. Allowing such an intimate part of your life to be on public display requires a lot of courage and I am deeply indebted to them all for their willingness to have their lives exposed in this way. Some of the individuals interviewed have preferred to remain anonymous; in these cases a pseudonym has been used to protect their identities.

Part II is devoted to an analysis of the experience of those interviewed in terms of the common elements they used to facilitate their own healing from serious illness. In order to highlight the different facets of this process I have grouped the common themes that emerge from their experience under a number of different chapter headings. These themes are applicable to the healing of all chronic diseases, including cancer, heart disease and stroke. It is hoped that readers will find this helpful in discerning some of the essential elements in how these people were able to transcend the bounds of what was thought to be possible.

In the collating and writing of this book I have been struck by profound correlations between the experiences of those interviewed and some of the tenets of healing systems I have studied over the years. As my understanding of health and disease has been largely informed by Ayurveda, the traditional system of medicine of India, and yoga, I introduce readers not familiar with these ancient systems of healing to some of their basic principles as seems pertinent.

In Part III I give readers some insights into how I have come to have such an interest in and commitment to complementary medicine. I also share some of my own experience of illness and the insights this experience has given me. In particular I look at my understanding of why I got sick and how I was able to facilitate the healing of an ulcerated and inflamed bowel condition.

This book is offered as a focus for reflection into the nature of healing, particularly for those with a personal experience of illness. It is hoped that wisdom gleaned from direct experience may serve to encourage more creative approaches to restoring wellbeing rather than be used as a recipe book for how to get well. Healing is necessarily a highly individual process and, in simple terms, what works for some will often not work for others. As such I would encourage readers to allow time for quiet contemplation of the stories contained in this book. Out of this may come a clearer idea of what actions need to be taken, what thoughts or attitudes need to be reconsidered or what feelings need to be expressed in order for healing to take place. On a professional level, it would be gratifying to think that the experiences shared in this book may go a little way to stimulating the hearts and minds of my colleagues.

Shaun Matthews
Sydney, 2002

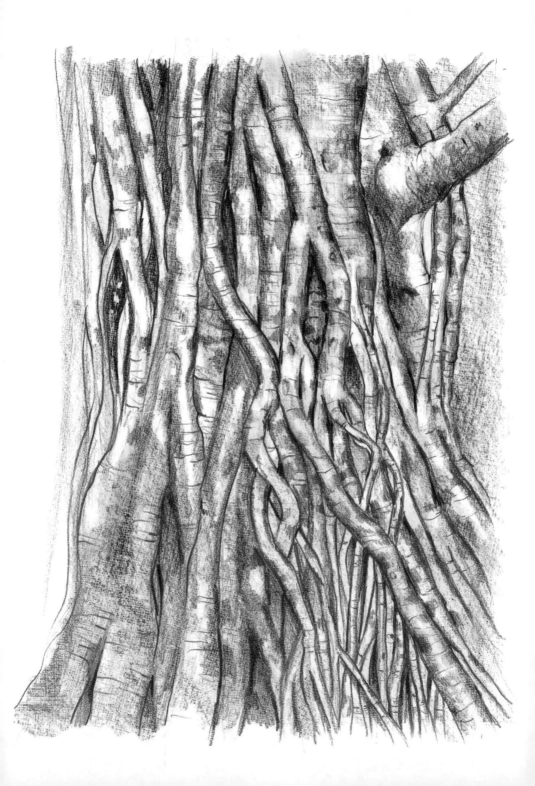

The Interviews

PART I

Roots of the Indian banyan tree, symbolising healing anchored in the substratum of human experience

Nicki's story

Born in 1962, Nicki Youdale was one of Australia's last thalidomide babies. Her mother had taken four tablets of thalidomide for morning sickness during the first term of her pregnancy. Thalidomide, available at that time without a prescription, was touted as a wonder drug and used in the treatment of nausea. As a result of her mother's ingestion of those four tablets Nicki suffers from a severe form of congenital heart disease and was also born without any thumbs.

I have known Nicki since childhood and saw her for the first time in several years in my consulting rooms because she was interested to learn more about Ayurveda as a healing science. Her story made a powerful and immediate impression on me, it was impossible not to feel privileged to be hearing her story and I felt that more people should be given the opportunity of hearing it. Accordingly, when the idea for this book first entered my mind I immediately thought of asking Nicki if she would agree to share her experiences with the general public, to which she generously obliged.

Nicki works part-time as a make-up artist and lives in the seaside Sydney suburb of Bondi. Nicki still has good days and bad days but has never given up her courageous attitude to the adversities life has confronted her with.

How did you first become aware that you were sick and how was it diagnosed?

I knew I was sick as a child, though I didn't really know what it was. I went to America to the Mayo Clinic and that's when the doctors discovered the hole in my heart. It had caused irreversible damage to the lungs so they couldn't repair the hole in the heart. For many years I was under the care of a paediatrician who kept refusing to do the test they did in America on me, which is to inject you with a dye and see how it goes round your system, because the paediatrician knew it would upset my mother too much. So he kept putting it off. I think he was concerned about my mother and didn't want her to know the full extent of the malformation, probably because he thought I was going to die as a child anyway. So why make her more concerned?

> 'I guess [my illness] made me pretty tough. I don't remember ever doing the "Why me?" syndrome. To me it was perfectly normal.'

All this came about because my mother walked into a chemist shop when she was 25 and pregnant with me, and said 'I can't sleep' or 'I don't feel well' and the chemist said, 'Take these four tablets and you'll be right.' Then the news broke in 1961 about the side effects of thalidomide. By that stage Mum was already pregnant and I was born in 1962. So I'm virtually one of the youngest.

I spent a lot of my childhood in hospital and I don't have a lot of memories of that except that there was always a nurse sitting next to me, close to my bed. I could never figure out why someone would sit there all night. I had lots of trips to hospital as a child. There used to be a bed in the staff room in junior school and I would invariably end up there having to sleep or lie down as I used to get migraines as a child and would go down in a screaming heap.

What were the symptoms you experienced when you were young?

As a baby I had projectile vomiting, my food couldn't pass down into my stomach, so Mum used to feed me sitting on the kitchen floor with a mop and bucket at the other end. Finally some doctor said to her, 'Just give her this to relax her muscles and she'll start gaining weight.'

As a child I just remember lots of stuffed toys in children's hospitals and hanging onto doctors' fingers while they were X-raying me, as I was so frightened of the machines. In those days it used to be huge, noisy machines so it was very scary.

I was always feeling tired and breathless and had lots of headaches. I used to get stomachaches and catch anything that was going around. Whichever child got the mumps or measles would pass it on to me. I had all those childhood diseases reoccur and it would take longer for my body to get over them. I was just a very weak, sick child. I couldn't do sport or anything like that and I remember being very lonely as a child, because I was either not at school enough to make solid friends or I'd get sick at lunchtime and have to go and lie down. Then I repeated a year and my best friend remembers my mother coming through the playground asking the girls in my year to play with me because I had no friends. I wasn't at school very much so I didn't know them and they didn't know me. They just knew me as the sick kid who wasn't picked for the sports teams.

How has your condition affected you in other ways? You've told me how it affected you physically, how did it affect you emotionally?

I guess it made me pretty tough. I don't remember ever doing the 'Why me?' syndrome. To me it was perfectly normal. I don't have memories of looking at other kids. Sure there were times when I thought, 'I wish I could play sport or have more friends' or something like that.

I think I probably also had a bit of anger that I took out on my poor mother because I would get sick so often at school, as I didn't like school. Everything there was an effort, all the classrooms were up a flight of stairs, so I was always the last one walking in, feeling a bit embarrassed. I think I coped as well as I could have given the circumstances. I used to get upset and I'd throw my suitcase at my mother or something like that.

But in saying all that I had a great network of friends as I got older who would say, 'Come on, Nick, we'll drag you up the stairs,' or 'Come on, Nick, we'll carry your bags to the next classroom.' Plus there was my sister Romaine. When I went to America for specialised medical tests I was six years old and she was four and I left here with long hair and looking the way I'd always looked to her and I came back with really short hair and was covered in scars where they'd injected all the dye under my arms or in my groin.

Romaine thought, 'Oh, my God, she's been violated,' because I looked so different. She made up her mind at the age of four that she had to protect me and she still is very much like that.

At different times you've been very sick and you've had relatively well periods. Can you tell me a bit about that?

It's been, on an average, two or three [hospital] admissions per year and then a couple of quick trips to the hospital for morphine for the angina I get or for a migraine that I just couldn't get rid of. There's been a lot of hospital and a lot of luck. There were times there when I shouldn't have gotten well and I did. Even [in the last decade], there were times when doctors were saying to me, 'You are losing the battle.' So they are all just as surprised as I am that I'm still here. But I think Lady Luck or someone has been on my side for sure.

You said that about ten years ago there was a significant change in your attitude to your illness?

Yeah, that came about because I started getting very weak and very breathless, I had a lot of angina and I went to see Dr Victor Chang [the late leading Sydney heart surgeon]. Funnily enough, when I was six years old at the Mayo Clinic in America, a young doctor said to Mum: 'Come the day they do heart and lung transplants, your daughter would need one but she probably won't live that long. But that's the kind of thing that would fix her condition.' That was the late Sixties and it was almost like saying: 'If we could get her to the moon and back she'll be okay.' So I couldn't get well, I had a lot less energy, lots of breathlessness and pain.

So we went to see Victor Chang and he said, 'Okay, we'll put you on the heart-lung transplant program.' I carried a beeper for ten months and would go into hospital for monthly visits so they could keep an eye on how I was going. I walked in there towards the end of the ten-month period and there were some recipients sitting waiting around to have their checkup. I took one look at them and absolutely flipped. I thought, 'God, you guys look worse than I do.' So I didn't even stay for my appointment, I just fled out of the hospital and went home. I was living with a really lovely guy and said to him: 'There's got to be another way. I've got to get well some other way. I'm not going to have this transplant, it just looks too scary.'

So we started doing the rounds of naturopaths and went down to Chinatown. You name it, I tried it. Nothing really worked. I was boiling up bark and drinking all this hideous stuff and it just wasn't happening. One day somebody said to me, 'Why don't you go down to see this extraordinary GP in Double Bay and see what he says?' I walked in there and said to him: 'You're my last chance.' And he said, 'Look, Nick, I don't think I can make you well enough to come off the waiting list but I can certainly strengthen your body so you can go through the transplant and have perhaps a better outcome than some of the people you saw in there.' I said, 'Okay, I'll try that, I'll settle for that.'

So he started me on a fairly strict vegetarian diet, I don't think I've ever juiced so many carrots in my life! Lots of vitamins at different intervals during the day and a lot of them were tissue repairers and good for heart maintenance like hawthorn and ginkgo, plus vitamin B injections to give me some more energy. And a month later I was fine and came off the waiting list and then had five years of really good health. Sure there were still hospital visits and dealing with my blood situation, which requires blood letting from time to time.

I had five years of good health and then I started going downhill again, but this time the breathlessness and pain and organ deterioration was a lot more severe. So I started having intravenous hydrogen peroxide, putting bleach into your veins, which worked for about three days and I would be back to being very breathless again. It was extremely painful to have it done because it comes straight out of the fridge and then goes into your veins, so I would have a really big head spin after it. But it did stop my organs – kidneys, liver and stomach – from being in so much pain because now they were getting some more oxygen. But as soon as it wore off, I was back to pain. It got to the stage when I couldn't really walk from here to there [pointing across the room] without being in a lot of pain and very, very breathless.

Then I had to get things like a home oxygen machine and we just started getting ready for my death. I started sorting papers and doing a will, this was in '95; '94 and '95 were the worst years. In 1995 we had what we thought was the final Christmas, which was the greatest Christmas I've ever had. There were a lot of old friends there and it was great! But I was very blue and very breathless and one night I remember glancing up into the mirror when I was studying and I was so blue and I stood up and went, 'Oh, God!' and could hardly breathe so I rang my best friend who just lives across the road. And she came flying over and burst into tears and said, 'Oh, I can't lose you; you can't die now. We've got to get you well.' And I said: 'Well, just call an ambulance for God's sake.'

There were lots of incidents like that; it was probably the worst year of my life. It was really tough; tough in terms of what my body was going through and the pain of that, but psychologically it was fairly peaceful. I thought: 'Okay, I'm dying,' and I was fine about that. 'There's going to be an end to the pain and trying to get up stairs and all that sort of stuff.' But dying takes a long time and I got very bored sitting on the couch and watching videos [laughing]. 'Come on, happen!' I got so bored that it actually propelled me into: 'What can I do to get well again?' So I started by being very strict with my diet again; not that I ever went off the bandwagon that much.

> 'I thought: "Okay, I'm dying," and I was fine about that. But dying takes a long time and I got very bored sitting on the couch and watching videos.'

Then I started having intravenous vitamin C in August 1996 and by late September I was fine. I was back to the health I have now. I got through the winter flu without going into hospital, which was just amazing. [The next year, as a protection against the flu] my doctor said, 'We are going to boost you with gamma globulin, vitamin B and vitamin C. So I thought: 'Great.' But you never know what it's going to be like from week to week. It's hard to plan your life and it gets a bit ... I wouldn't say I get pissed off. I get really scared whenever I have to confront this transplant thing again, that absolutely terrifies me. It really does. That's where the child in me says: 'Wow, this is all too scary.' The big machines, like the big X-ray machines that they used to have. It all gets too daunting.

It goes back to those memories as a child?

Yes, exactly. It's too much, it gets really scary and I go into denial. I can't think too much about the whole thing. Luckily I've had a terrific family and great friends who have supported me, especially since 1995 when I organised our high-school reunion. Now every month, as a spin off of that, we have what's called 'The Nicki Dinners'. We go round to one of the girls' places for dinner. They started it because some of my girlfriends said. 'Nicki is dying, let's do something for her, let's have a special dinner for her once every now and then.'

Then I got well and I said, 'Can we still keep the dinners going?' [laughing] and they said, 'Yes, of course!' Now we refer to them as 'The Girlie Dinners'. The great thing was they've all been able to link up too because almost all of them, except two of us, are mothers. So they now have their mothers' group and all that sort of stuff together too. It's been a great opportunity for everyone to reconnect since school days. Even though I organised the whole reunion, because I was so ill I was the last one to get there and the first to leave. I don't really remember that night very well at all, except for slamming down two daiquiris and that was about it!

So I guess it has been a roller coaster. [One day a few months ago] I woke up and I was ready to cut my left arm off I was in so much pain. 'Shit, I've got angina again! And badly.' So I rang a girlfriend, because I couldn't find anyone else family wise, and she took me into the hospital. I had angina from dehydration. I can go from being quite well to 24 hours later, saying to myself, 'Shit! What's happening?'

A lot of uncertainty?

Always. Do I start a course? And if I get sick am I going to be able to catch up? So my life has been a stop-start with courses and with jobs. I have to knock back certain jobs because I can't continue to work. I worked on a film a couple of weeks ago for the Tropicana Film Festival and that involved a twelve-hour shooting day. I was fine right through that day but the next day I couldn't speak. Then I was offered a feature film last week and I had to turn it down. I could do four, five or six days of those hours for six weeks. It's a bit annoying.

Last year, I can't believe it, I actually managed to finish a course, which was the Lifeline telephone counselling course. So now I'm on the phone as a counsellor, which is great. But it was a huge achievement in terms of, 'Yes, I actually finished a course!' For the first time in many, many years. It was great! I met some fabulous people. But yeah, it's still a roller coaster.

What have been some of the positive aspects of being ill, having had this experience of illness for so long?

I guess when you get a handle on ... and I don't think anyone has a handle on it one hundred percent, when you get to a space where you feel more at ease about your mortality. And you can then put that aside and say, 'Okay, now what can I do? So that's going to happen to everyone, it may happen to me a little sooner. What can I do so that between now and then I can have some fun?' Because in '95 when I was quite ill and was getting close [to death], the only thing you remember are the good times in life. You don't remember the fight you had with your mother or something stupid or the broken hearts you've had over the years or whatever. You just remember the really fun things you did.

'[Close to death] you don't remember the fight with your mother or the broken hearts over the years. You just remember the fun things.'

So I guess where I come from now is, I really just want to enjoy as much as I can and have some fun and just be around people. Not only that, having my condition, it's allowed me to meet some really extraordinary people, and get to know them. The lung physician on the transplant team is one of the most amazing men I have ever met.

A girlfriend of mine is a strict Buddhist and she said to me, 'I've just been on a retreat with this Tibetan Rimpoche [high priest] and I've told him all about you. They want to give you a blessing. I said [chuckling], 'Okay, when am I getting this blessing?' She said, 'You have to be at Sydney airport when they fly out.' It was extraordinary. Here was this Tibetan monk with the face of a thousand lives, an extraordinary looking man, with his hands on my head giving me a blessing. And saying, 'You should have the operation, and look after your diet,' all that sort of stuff. So experiences like that have just been incredible.

People are very caught up in always wanting to appear as if their lives are good or as if there's no illness in the family. Everyone is so guarded about talking about someone's condition in the family or a death in the family. But if I'm talking to someone and I say, 'Yes, I can understand how upsetting it must be for you to deal with your sick child because I have lived that life,' it cuts down a lot of barriers and you really get to talk to people on a very honest level, from a really grounded point as opposed to just the pleasantries of conversation. With a lot of my friends the conversation is not a case of, 'Don't worry, Nick, you will be right,' which is the last thing you want to hear. It's: 'God, that must be really hard for you.'

I've met a lot of people I probably wouldn't have met had I been well. One of my most prominent memories is of Christmas in '94; I was in hospital with ruptured stomach ulcers and septicaemia. Also I had had a minor stroke when I was in there on Boxing Day. I am always on the cardiac ward and all the other patients are quite elderly, so there's rarely anyone to really talk to. Two rooms down from me was a young girl of my age, an Aborigine who was a street worker and was in hospital for exactly the same thing as me. There's this image of us that I keep remembering, we both had our little drip trolleys and were pacing the hallway. And we live worlds apart, our realities are very different and yet we just had the best conversations about life and whatever else. It doesn't matter what your upbringing is, when you've got a common disease or something like that, no matter how much love or money you have, it's not going to make it better. So it was just extraordinary, to spend five weeks in hospital with this girl. Because we couldn't sleep, we just paced the corridors with our drip stands talking about life. It was amazing. I often wonder what happened to her. I'll have to take a drive one evening.

Having a condition, you don't suffer fools gladly. My best friend said if her husband comes out and complains to her of a sore foot or something like that, she says, 'Don't even think it or even talk to me about your sore foot. Look what Nicki goes through.' And he says to me, 'Do you realise, Nicki, I can't get away with anything now because of you!' [laughing].

It's been a very unusual life and I've had many wonderful gifts in terms of friendships and people I've met. It's funny, in the last few months my life has changed enormously, dealing with being ill and getting well and trying to stay well. Then dealing with the question of whether to have a heart-lung transplant and trying to get the courage up to say, 'Yes, I will have it.' And walking into the hospital and the doctors saying, 'Sorry, you're too ill.'

And with all that, still dealing with the blood problems and breathlessness and the oxygen machine ... So some wonderful gifts have happened to me in my life and it's been great. It's also been very lonely; it's also been really scary. I guess I don't get so obsessed by the silly little things in life. I mean, sure I do, we are all human, but they don't rule my life where sometimes they rule other people's lives, like how they look or 'Am I driving the right car?'. It doesn't matter how much money you spend, at the end of the day you are still going to be scattered or buried, one or the other.

Where would you say you get your strength from?

My sisters, Romaine and Manon, and my friends. My mother and father have had a huge influence on me and in many ways have the same outlook on life. My father went through the war and saw his close friends die and I guess it just gives you a better understanding and an outlook where you don't take too much for granted, because it can all be taken away from you. Dad and I have had great conversations about the philosophical side of life. Also I've got a lot of strength from my mother, who was only 25 when she gave birth to me in the Sixties. People said, 'Oh, God, look at that baby and that terrible woman who took those drugs.' She coped with all that, with the support of my father. As I said to her, that is obviously where I learnt some strategies on how to cope. She said, 'Well, I go numb sometimes, that's how I cope,' and I said, 'Yeah, so do I, you just go numb.'

I think also you've got to have a sense of humour because if you don't have a sense of humour it just gets so depressing. There's nothing like a good laugh, laughing is the best medicine, it really is. That's where I got my strength from, a combination of family, friends and being pig-headed and determined that even though I had this condition, I still wanted to do what my other friends were doing. I made a choice not to buy into the condition and live the condition, which would make me a crashing bore because it bores the hell out of me.

Not only that, someone said to me regarding all the hospital visits, 'How do you cope with your life being so exposed?' I've grown up with medical students all my life around the bed saying, 'Great clubbing!' or 'Did you hear the so-and-so sound in the heart beat?' I went through my teenage years and twenties and thirties, stripped to the waist, with a lot of medical students standing around my bed. Every part of my life has been exposed. So I guess I'm used to having my whole life being on display. It teaches you not to get too precious about a few things.

Nicki, what are the things you've done that have helped facilitate your healing?

Buteyko breathing has definitely helped, which was developed by a Russian doctor who was working with people who were in the process of dying. He noticed that they all hyperventilated, which seemed to expedite their death. So he came up with a breathing technique which involves a series of pauses in the breath, followed by shallow breathing for two or three minutes and then another pause. You increase the carbon dioxide in your blood so when you breathe in you can utilise the oxygen a lot better. I do that every morning and I should do it every night, but I'm a bit slack sometimes [chuckling].

You know when you wake up in the morning and you're a bit groggy and it takes a little while to get the senses together; two pauses with two minutes of breathing and bang, you're awake! You feel so alive it's amazing! That's helped enormously. It's also helped with my blood circulation, my legs and feet used to ache enormously every night and now they don't at all. It's increased my energy level a lot, before I used to drive down to Bondi Beach just to have a walk. Now I can walk there, have a walk on the beach and then walk back. I sleep better. It curbs your eating. You only really eat when you're hungry, so you're not just doing the old comfort food routine. It's had an enormous effect. And if I don't do it, the nurse that gives me intravenous vitamin C once a week, who is also a Buteyko practitioner, can spot it straightaway. She'll say, 'Look how much more fluid you're retaining, look how blue you are, how much more bloated in the face you are.' Then she'll say, 'Don't worry, in four days you'll be back to normal.' Which is great, it really keeps me on track.

So the other thing is the intravenous vitamin C, I have 15 grams of that a week, which only stays in your body 24–36 hours but it re-energises every cell in your body and has a lasting effect for close to a week. I made the mistake of going for thirteen days over the Christmas break without it and paid the price. I wound up on the oxygen machine for two days, very breathless, very tired and so it took 30 grams of intravenous C over two days to get me back on track. So without it I'd be in big trouble, really big trouble.

I also take a number of prescription drugs such as a very mild heart drug, fluid retention tablets, migraine tablets, aspirin, warfarin, potassium supplements and a whole heap of vitamins, and have a basically vegetarian diet.

> 'I made a choice not to buy into and live the condition, which would make me a crashing bore because it bores the hell out of me.'

Having had all of this experience, how do you understand the process of healing?

You've got to want to get better because it doesn't really matter what you do, if you don't mentally want to get well, you won't get well. Or you will for a little while. My experience was that I was so frightened of going through the transplant that I was completely dedicated to finding an alternative route.

From what you've said before, it sounds like you were more frightened of having the heart-lung transplant than of dying?

Yeah, absolutely, without a doubt. Dying to me is the end of pain, it's the end of drugs, it's the end of needles, the end of uncertainty and it's peaceful. The thought of going through the transplant then having to cope with all the drugs post-transplant ... and not only that, the transplant signifies to me the beginning of the end. There is only a certain amount of years that I will live after the transplant. It could be five, it could be ten, maybe I can live for fifteen years, I don't know. It depends on how good the match is and the problems I have after the heart-lung transplant.

You get very used to what your organs can and can't do, whereas after the transplant it will be a whole new ball game. But in saying all that I am ready to go on the waiting list, if in the next year or two my health situation changes. But for now it's great.

You look great.

Actually, I've got a shocking hangover; I went to a wedding over the weekend and a big party yesterday! The great thing is I can do things like that. It will take me two days to really feel a lot better whereas before I just couldn't. Yes, I'm very strict with my diet but it comes to a point where you think, 'Oh, to hell with it, give me some more champagne!'

You need to take control psychologically and get proactive, because a lot of people live in denial, and die in denial. And take the attitude, 'I'll be right, don't worry.' Then suddenly they go to the doctor and the doctor says: 'You're riddled with cancer. You've got a month to live.' And people usually do live right to that date.

As I've always said: 'Don't put your head in the sand, get proactive.' If you don't ask, if you're not in the conversation of life ... Life is not stingy; people are stingy. But when you get in and say, 'Now I want to try something,' you've really got to get very proactive because no-one else is going to do it for you.' I didn't even tell my parents I was going to try all this alternative stuff. I didn't tell anyone and then when I said, 'I'm off the transplant list,' people would respond, 'What do you mean you're going off the transplant list?' They were in shock, they couldn't believe it and had I have waited or not had the guts to say to myself: 'Well, fuck it, what have I got to lose?' then I probably would have been dead by now, without a doubt. But I guess it was fear that got me to be very proactive in my life in looking after myself. So, fear is a very good thing! [laughing lightly].

A strong motivator.

It is a huge motivator, absolutely.

How did you manage financially through all of this?

Well, all thalidomide affected people were compensated and you were compensated to the degree of your disability or deformity. Now, that wasn't very much money. Back in the Sixties and Seventies when they were working it out it certainly sounded like a lot of money but it wasn't very much money really. I have survived as a freelance make-up artist for most of my life, as well as doing things like reception jobs. In 1996 I finally succumbed and applied for the disability pension, which is now my main form of income.

So money hasn't been flowing, but being a make-up artist, when I work it pays very well. I've also done other little jobs like receptioning, little jobs that keep me going. Lots of weddings, working on weekends. At times it has been pretty tough and my parents have been very supportive, which has been great. But once you've paid for a week of alternative medicine, which costs me roughly one hundred dollars a week just to stay well, there's not a whole lot left in the kitty to go and splurge. I pay great homage to the lay-by god, I buy everything on lay-by! That's the way you live, there's no holidays or expensive things like that but every now and then, like last year when I started to get well, I just loaded up the car and disappeared to Byron Bay for a month.

I was fed up with doctors and hospitals and the whole bit, so I put my oxygen machine in the car and just disappeared. It was great! So doing things like that has probably saved my sanity, though my mother will respond with: 'What if you get sick up there and something happens?' Well I say, 'I get sick up there and something happens.' I can't live worried about it. Mum worries about that sort of stuff and I say, 'Well, I don't have to worry about it 'cause you are. So I'll go and have a good time.'

> *Well said! [laughing together] I also wanted to ask what advice would you give to other people facing serious or life-threatening illness?*

Get proactive. You have to fall in love with your disease to a degree, so that it doesn't become something that you leave in the too-hard basket. You have to keep talking to people, keep on asking questions, try different things. Just get proactive, because if you don't, nothing against doctors, but they have workloads that are huge. Unless you are in there asking the questions, at the end of the day no-one really gives a damn about you. They do, but not to the same degree. If you don't take charge and get proactive and look after yourself, then you'll have a lot of people turning up at your funeral saying how fabulous you were! [chuckling together] And your funeral may be a little sooner than it could have been!

In many ways it's a lot more difficult for women because you have certain images cast upon you by society; what you should look like, all that body image stuff. Women, for example, who've had a mastectomy have to deal with: 'Oh, God, I don't look like a woman any more.' I only use that reference in terms of when I found out I couldn't have children, the last thing you feel like is a feminine woman, you feel like no-man's-land. It's like: 'You mean I can't have children? I'm a woman! There's biological things going off in me, gongs ticking away.'

I really got confronted with that when my best friend had her two children. I couldn't walk into the hospital. I was just a basket case. Then I made myself do it a few days later just to see her babies. If you bind to the negativity of, 'Okay, I can't have children,' or 'I've lost my breast through cancer and I don't feel like a woman;' if you bind to that conversation and stay in that conversation, then the only thing that will happen is that evidence will keep coming up reaffirming that in your mind. 'No man will ever be attracted to me because of my heart condition or because I can't have children.' Well, if I kept that in place then that would be my reality.

I'm not saying it's easy not to have that in place. Sometimes you do buy into the whole thing and it gets really depressing. In '97 I was really well for the first time in many years and single, sitting at home Saturday night after Saturday night with a video and saying to myself: 'Nicki, get a life for God's sake.' If you have trouble dealing with certain things about health or whatever, don't keep it to yourself. Go and talk to professionals and shop around until you find the best psychologist, psychiatrist, friend, whatever. Don't keep it to yourself. Everything is much better out than in, don't store the tears up, don't store the anger up, don't store the fear up. Just get it out, because if it stays inside it will kill you before your disease does. Or drive you to kill yourself, one way or the other. You only get one shot at life, that's what a lot of people forget.

In many ways I'm very grateful for the great gifts that my life has given me; the very special people in it. Okay, it's not the life I thought I was going to have when I left school, which was to get married and have kids and all that stuff. It has taken some adjusting and talking to people, but all in all, hospital visits, everything included, it's been a good life, a really good life. Being in my thirties I must say I'm enjoying it a hell of a lot more, ever since I took control of my health.

A turning point?

A huge turning point and that's what I say to anyone, if you really want to have the opportunity to experience some lovely things in your life, you're not going to do it unless you do the hard work first, and the hard work is bloody hard. It's really scary sometimes and it's really lonely, you get really pissed off. But if you're courting death, and I have been [my whole life], you need to get a handle on it. I see it as the end of the pain ... and peace. I would rather have a short good life than a dragged out one.

'If you have trouble dealing with certain things about health, don't keep it to yourself ... get it out, because it will kill you before your disease does.'

Rebecca's story

*I*t was while Rebecca was au pairing in France in 1988 that she first heard from an American woman of a condition called myalgic encephalomyelitis (ME), another name for chronic fatigue syndrome (CFS). She recognised the symptoms. Rebecca was twenty at the time and though her energy often allowed her to participate in life in a very full way, it hadn't been stable since she'd had a viral infection in her final year of school in 1984.

Rebecca's health declined while staying in the United Kingdom and she decided to return home to Australia. Over the next four years her health continued to follow a pattern of high energy (in which periods she undertook many work and creative activities) followed by months of exhaustion and excessively low energy. A prolonged course of Chinese herbs prescribed by a practitioner of Traditional Chinese Medicine brought considerable improvement, though her health seriously relapsed four years later. This time the pattern broke. Months passed and she didn't recover her energy. In 1993, chronic fatigue syndrome was eventually diagnosed and Rebecca set about the task of healing herself.

I met Rebecca in 1997 when she invited me to talk at a one-day seminar on Ayurvedic and yogic approaches to managing low-energy conditions. During the seminar Rebecca shared her own hard-won experience about which approaches to healing had helped her over the years. I could not help but be impressed by the wisdom in her words and felt that she would make a wonderful contribution to this book. Rebecca shares generously what it is like to have chronic fatigue syndrome and her understanding of the healing process.

What was the nature of your illness and how was it diagnosed?

Well, to talk about the nature of it without calling it anything, I became increasingly tired in a way I hadn't been tired before. It seemed a different sort of tiredness; it wasn't the tiredness you have after a late night.

It felt different?

It did, it felt really deep within my body. At the time it didn't seem to come from anything I was doing. I didn't actually get sick (in terms of the usual viral infection) at the time that I came into this deep part of the illness. That is, I was just getting more and more tired. I was working towards the idea of resigning from work and going travelling to India. So I had this idea that when I finished work things would improve.

> 'It was like the tiredness and the tears were coming from somewhere I didn't know about yet.'

I was seeing a Chinese doctor at the time and I kept saying to him, 'Look, I'm just getting more and more tired, I think something is seriously wrong with me.' And he always used to say to me, 'Yes, your system is so down, you've burnt very brightly, you're going to take a long time to recover.' This was way before anything.

Then it started that I would have to go and lie down during the day. I had never done that in my life, so it was something that was quite hard for my pride as well. I saw myself as someone who didn't lie down in the middle of the day [laughing]. I had all these kinds of standards. I remember one incident when I was out with my partner in a CD shop and I was interested in looking at CDs but I felt myself fading. I said, 'I think I'm going to have to go home and lie down.' It was really strange. He was really shocked too because we were really pretty 'gung ho'.

The other thing that started happening was that I would wake up in the morning and I wouldn't have gained anything from sleep. I'd wake up to get ready for work and I'd just feel this absolute exhaustion in my body. I started to get really teary and I remember a few mornings just crying and that felt really strange as well. It was like the tiredness and the tears were coming from somewhere that I didn't know about yet. I can't really explain it any better than that. It was like I was crying before I had thought about anything. I guess there was a feeling of losing control. I'd keep praying then get ready and go off to work. That's how it came on. I had about a month before I was due to end work and I was increasingly tired and struggling at work. I was a book editor in a publishing company, which was really intense work where you are concentrating all day and looking closely at things and having to make really important decisions. And I was feeling less and less able to and that was freaking me out.

I'd be at work and the whole time everyone was asking me, 'How is your trip for India working out?' And I just played into the whole thing, and yet inside I was freaking out because something was wrong with me but I didn't feel I could tell anyone. So I'd say, 'Oh, yeah, we've got a guidebook and we're doing this and this, and this is what's going to happen.'

I kept going and seeing my doctor and saying, 'I'm not getting any better. Something is happening.' He'd moved practice. It used to be across the road and now I had to get the train and walk up this hill to get to his practice. It was a real struggle walking up the hill and I was a real walker. I loved walking. I used to walk everywhere. So that was really frightening. It doesn't seem so bizarre to me now; it's normal. But it wasn't normal then and I was thinking, 'What is wrong with me? This hill is really small, something's going on.' I'd get there and I just felt something was going on which was much bigger than what even he was seeing. Although I trusted that he was treating me in the way he could and giving me stuff to help me.

When I finished work I thought, 'Now it will go away.' But the day after I left work I couldn't get out of bed. It was just like I'd completely shut down. In that week I had done something stupid. I'd gone and had my shots for India and that had wiped me out. So for two weeks I just couldn't do much. I could just walk to the shop at the end of the street and I wouldn't be able to get home. This kind of crazy stuff. That's when you begin to panic and start to come up with all these ideas about what one should do. I went up to this place in the mountains, where a friend had a house. I was up there on my own and that was a really confronting week. I just realised that I couldn't do much. I didn't have a phone at the house and my partner had asked me to ring him to tell him if I was okay. So I had to walk a couple of kilometres to a public phone. I'll never forget that walk. It was just the most awful thing. I had to walk a bit then sit down. It was quite an isolated place and by the time I got to the phone I was in tears. It was like a complete not knowing; not knowing what's going on and I'd started to panic.

That time is really blurry now. I kept going back to my Chinese doctor. He had a different perspective. He wasn't going to name my illness. I think I wanted [it to be named], I wanted something tangible. So I started to tell him that and he said, 'Go and see my wife who practises Western medicine.' So I went and saw her and she said, 'You're a classic case of chronic fatigue syndrome, that's what it is.' And it was like, 'Great! It's something!' But then you realise that that doesn't mean anything. I was at point A again. But that was my diagnosis, to answer your question.

How has it affected you having chronic fatigue syndrome up to this point?

Where to begin? [laughing loudly]! Obviously there's just a dramatic lifestyle change, but it didn't happen straightaway because for a long time, and certainly at the beginning, there was a complete fighting against it, not wanting that unknown thing to take over my life. So I didn't change my lifestyle enough, which probably was calling for a dramatic change. I wasn't emotionally or psychically ready for that. So, I went back to work instead of going to India. I took on part-time work and really I was so unwell then and doing that work was just crazy.

I guess the worst parts about that first stage were really not knowing what was wrong with me and not being able to articulate that to anyone else. So therefore not getting much support, I didn't feel supported at all except by my partner who supported me enormously. But my family and friends were saying things like, 'Maybe you should do some exercise.' I had been a really fit person, so that didn't make sense to me. Nothing was making sense. I didn't really know where else to get support.

That was the early days of chronic fatigue syndrome, then?

Yes, people had not heard of it.

It was still a relatively unknown entity.

People were just beginning to talk about it. In fact I had a couple of friends who were psychiatric nurses who I was out with one night and they were saying, 'Have you heard about this new thing people are getting?' And I was going, 'Oh, actually …' [nervous laugh]. I couldn't tell people because I didn't even know if I believed it myself. I had this whole crazy thing in my head about it.

As far as lifestyle changes go, prior to that time I was doing fairly strenuous yoga, I was going to the gym, on weekends we used to climb mountains, go bushwalking. My partner was really into rock climbing and I had started to learn. We were really pretty active and very active socially as well. I tried to keep all of that up for a while and I had some pretty horrible experiences of being really caught out with that stuff.

Eventually I had to stop work and I decided to move interstate to work on a writing project. I thought to myself, 'I'll just do what makes me happy and that will work.' So I did this month of writing intensely with someone, and that was really good but it was just pumping up my adrenal glands. I was drinking lots of coffee and going for it. At the end of that I was probably worse. I moved to the mountains and even then endeavoured to get more work until I came to a point that I had to stop. Everything stopped and that's probably when it had got to a point where I knew that some major things had to change. So stopping work was a really big one for me, a really big one. That was a major change.

I also had to give up the exercise I enjoyed like bushwalking and yoga. I just lived for these things. The yoga was really interesting because yoga, I'd believed, was meant to make you strong and healthy. This presented a major conflict for me because I was reading the texts and seeing what yoga was meant to be doing and it wasn't happening for me. I was doing yoga and it was wiping me out. So that became a real struggle and something that I had to let go of. That is I had to let go of the way I had been 'doing yoga' and to learn more about what yoga really was and not what we'd appropriated it as being. Through this I had to recognise my investment in everything being the way I wanted it to be.

Another big change was in my social life because I really love people and being with people. But again I think there was this investment in getting feedback about who I was through these interactions. I was starting to question all that and starting to realise that a lot of the socialising I'd been doing was making me tired. I just couldn't keep up with it all. The people in my world met for coffee and talked about their work and the latest films they'd seen. Conversation and ultimately ways of being with people obviously has to dramatically change if your lifestyle changes. I found I didn't have a lot to say any more. My experience seemed really full and really intense but I'd be in situations where I felt it wasn't really appropriate to talk about that stuff. It didn't feel like it was anyway.

> 'Previously I'd been with people who were robust and I wanted to be robust as well. I didn't want to know the people who weren't; I didn't want to be an "ill person."'

So I found that difficult and there was a lifestyle change as far as the types of people I felt comfortable with. I started meeting people who, I reflect now, were probably more willing to show their vulnerabilities. Previously I'd been with people who were much more robust and I guess I wanted to be robust as well. I didn't want to know the people who weren't, which was quite a confronting thing to come to as well. I didn't want to be an 'ill person'.

When I moved out of the city I was invited by someone to a support group for people with life-threatening and chronic illnesses. Although I was feeling very isolated, I remember feeling confronted by this invitation. One of the reasons was that I felt my illness wasn't as worthy as people in the group who had illnesses like cancer and AIDS. But the other thing was, I realise now, I just didn't want to be associated with people who were weak, who weren't coping. There was a real judgement in me that has probably contributed to and been tied up with the illness as well.

So your illness is weakness?

Yes, that was how I saw it then. Weakness, definitely. And I didn't want to be a weak person. I wanted to be a strong person. So if I'm with them, what does that mean? Yes, that has been a real change.

What happens to weak people?

Well, survival of the fittest. They don't survive in our society. I mean, they ultimately have to drop out and create their own society. Because if I compare what I have now to the world that I was in before, there was not a lot of space for it. There was not a lot of space for vulnerability.

In terms of the emotional effects of the illness, I felt 'undone' by it. It was like everything I thought I was was being unravelled. Like this wool I just kept pulling and pulling and everything I wanted to hold onto, in terms of physical things like work as well as other metaphysical ideas about who I was, my identity, my judgements, my opinion, my world-view, I could see it all unravelling. I was trying to hold onto something, 'cause when it's all going you don't know what's going to be left, because you think what's being unravelled is you.

I wasn't depressed originally. It actually took a few years for depression to kick in. It was more a whole process of hope and frustration, hope and frustration. This was the pattern. The illness hasn't been constant, I've actually felt I was getting better and then I've relapsed a number of times. I'm in my longest period now of no relapse and I believe that I'm out of it. There is a cyclical thing and when that happens a number of times it leads to despair. I think it happened a number of times and it led to depression. But that took a long time; I was very optimistic against quite severe odds. I maintained my optimism but was very weepy.

The biggest emotional effect was that feeling of being vulnerable, I felt like this naked self wondering how I'd survive in the world if I had nothing to protect me, not having all those masks and identities. How would I survive? So there's a real feeling of vulnerability. Whenever I get sick now, if I get a sore throat for a day, this huge emotion comes up in me and I associate it with that time of being vulnerable. That whole fear and sadness of not knowing what's happening and not being able to have power and to be able to cope in life.

Because it's been there so often in the past that now when you have physical symptoms it's like it's there again.

Straightaway! I have to work with it as soon as it comes. I have to say to myself: 'No, it's okay, this is what it is and maybe it's a cold and it will pass.' I need to do this immediately because I find I can go into a spiral quite fast.

It's hard to stay in the here and now.

Yes, for sure.

How are you at present?

I consider myself to be really well at present. It's been about four years now, so I can't really remember what 'well' meant. For myself there's all these definitions of wellness. The fact that I became so sick makes me question how really well I was, emotionally. I don't mean I was sick emotionally but I think I had some pretty strong patterns of behaviour and thinking, things that were really weakening my immune system. Interestingly enough the patterns were based on maintaining robustness of character and being perceived that way and wanting to be strong in the world. I actually think that ironically that whole thing was weakening me.

So now I'm quite well, I still have to adhere to certain rules and regulations in my life. I'm much more flexible than I was even six months ago, but I have to do that to maintain this wellness. If too many of those slip, I can feel myself going down and I have to be really conscious of that. I can't live carelessly and that's really hard, because although people might think it would be great to live this healthy kind of life, it feels like a limitation. There's this part of me that just wants to break out! It's been a really strong part of me, but the part of me that broke out over the years got me in trouble, physically.

What did you do to break out?

Oh, I don't know, just went dancing or went for a rigorous bushwalk, stayed up late, stuff like that. I had such detrimental effects from coffee and alcohol, for example, that I had to stop consuming those immediately. Sometimes I want to break out so strongly, like go dancing, I'll dream about that because I used to love dancing. I just can't handle it any more. But at the moment I just feel really grateful because I can do things. This morning I went for a 40-minute walk, which I couldn't have done two years ago. I feel grateful a lot of the time, which is nice but it's a laugh really [laughing lightly], feeling grateful for such small things. It's really nice talking to other people who have been through the same thing because we can share things like, 'Isn't it amazing to just go to the shops and not think about the walk? To just go to the shops.'

Yes, such a simple thing.

So now I'm pretty well as long as I keep to my rules. The other thing is that if I get stress in my life, and I've had a bit lately, I just see the patterns, the old patterns in my nature. It's still so strong. I see an anxiety and it builds and I don't know how to deal with it, so I get really busy. I can feel that unravelling again, I'm being unravelled. The next thing I'm depleted. That can be from stress and from seeing too many people.

So I really enjoy people now, it's a lovely thing to be with people again and be able to feel I can be with them without it being too painful in a way. It used to be a bit painful to be with people. If I'm with people too much I will come home and feel really exhausted. I went home at Christmas to spend time with my family and friends and I think I was there for three weeks and it was just a week too much; too much talking, too much interacting, too much engaging. I have been taking Chinese herbs constantly and I don't know how I'd be if I wasn't.

I think you touched on this before but I was wondering, how do you understand why you got sick?

It's a hard question. It's hard to come to what you know, as opposed to what paradigms you have adopted. How cluttered you can become with all the theories and explanations for everything, for illness particularly, which abound at the moment. I went through different theories but what I think I came to (and I think I've been really influenced by

Ayurveda because it struck a chord) is that I have a particular predisposition to be a certain way.

I really understand my nature a bit more, what I'm like, how I react, what happens, who I am in the world and why, and am beginning to understand my motivations for being a certain way.

Then there is this other thing that happened when I was seventeen. I got some illness that affected my immune system and after that time I seemed to catch viruses and infections very easily, whereas I wasn't an unwell child. So I have this idea that it's my nature to be a certain way but my immune system has been damaged, which has exacerbated the problem. So that's my understanding. I think my nature and my tendencies, how I am emotionally in the world, has exacerbated this immune system problem or perhaps created it in the first place.

There are lots of other levels to speak on I guess. Sometimes there is this understanding, and I say this with caution, that it was my saving grace that this thing came along to help me not be as I was. I felt like I was in control then and am not in control now. But in another way I'm much more in control, because I know who I am. Whereas before I was operating in the world through these unconscious predispositions, 'I've got to do this, this and this.' I didn't have much of an idea or willingness to look at why I felt I needed to fill every second of the day.

> *'I was always a thinker, that's why I think it's a gift that this has happened to me. If it hadn't, who would I be? Where would I be going now?'*

So through the process you've become a more conscious person?

Yes, definitely. I was never completely unconscious. I was always a thinker, that's why I think it's a gift really, that this has happened to me, because if it hadn't happened, who would I be? Where would I be going now? I've got a better grip on that now.

There is, however, a possibility for that to be taken the wrong way. If someone tells you that being sick is a gift when you are just becoming ill, you just say, 'That's bullshit. I don't want to be sick.' I don't want to speak of illness as a gift without really acknowledging the pain and the struggle that this has meant; the extreme sadness and grief at losing things that I felt I was meant to be doing in my life. So I always want to acknowledge that simultaneously with saying, 'I'm glad for the results, but perhaps could I have a different journey next time?'

There's been a lot of loss.

Yes, there's been a lot of grief. I found grief was a major thing for a while but at least when I hit grief I knew that I had to be grieving.

What have been some of the most difficult things about being sick?

One thing that was difficult was relationships and feeling like you need special treatment. Needing people to acknowledge what's going on for you so that they can support you and at the same time feeling isolated because of that or feeling a burden on people. The difficulty of not knowing how to express those needs just made me pull away from people. It was just too hard with people without setting the rules or saying, 'I can only talk for half an hour' or 'Can I go and lie down?' or 'Can we not eat dinner at nine o'clock at night?' There was a whole lot of stuff I had to negotiate when being with people; especially with younger people, like myself. I found people unsupportive, though I think it was partly my fault for not actually expressing my needs. I would find people oblivious to my needs and that was really hard.

Another thing that was difficult was not knowing how to be sick. No-one tells you how to be sick. All of a sudden it's like you've got this new job and there's no guidelines, there's just nothing. I didn't know what to do with my days. I was seeing a doctor who is also a yoga therapist at that stage, which was helpful in so many ways, but still I'd come home and go, 'Yeah, but what the fuck do I do from nine to five? I'm just with myself.'

People would say, 'What do you do?' And I would say, 'I just spend the day doing a bit of reading then I rest.' You try to make it sound as okay as possible because you don't want people to feel sorry for you. 'Well, actually, it was hideous.' So they would say, 'Oh, that sounds great.' I got that a lot and I felt like saying, 'Well, actually, it's great to be at home and to rest and read a book. But it's not great when you don't know what's going to happen to you and you don't know if it's going to get worse or you're going to be like this for the rest of your life.' People like staying at home and reading when they know it's actually a break, an intermission between things, not when it's possibly permanent.

Not being able to do little things that you would like to do was difficult. I'd have these ideas about going to the shops and having a coffee just to change the scenery. I'd get up there and I'd find myself feeling incredibly vulnerable because I wasn't well. I could see myself trying to do these things and it made me really sad to see myself trying to cope. All that leads to this real feeling of isolation with what you're experiencing, not being able to explain things to people and therefore feeling more and more that you are retreating, retreating.

That there is an abyss between you and others.

Yes.

So what have been the most positive things about being sick?

I think it's been humbling, really humbling, and ultimately it's a damned fine thing to realise you're human; that we are all struggling with our various stuff. I think I've always been a very sympathetic person, but perhaps not empathetic. I think I did see a difference between myself and other people. I'd pity people who might be struggling rather than feel true empathy for them and true compassion.

Around financial matters as well, I believed that if you want money, you just go and get a job. I always felt secure in the fact that I had resources and the experience of being sick really shattered that. All of a sudden I didn't have them. I had to be dependent on the government for a while and I had to be dependent on other people for different things.

Before when I saw people's pain I think I wanted to save them, but when I got really close to their pain I felt really confronted by it. I didn't really want to know about it, I felt almost repulsed sometimes by people's pain. I lived with someone once who had chronic fatigue syndrome, who was really sick and depressed and I felt quite repulsed. I didn't want to be around her because it was really confronting. I find with people now, I can see their pain and it's no big deal. It is a big deal but I've got space for it. I think you do create space.

I went and saw Petrea King [a nurse, naturopath and fully recovered cancer patient who works with people who are facing life-threatening illness] speak once and she said something that really touched me; that really resonated. She said that your ability to be with other people's pain is dependent on your ability to feel your own pain. I thought that's really true. You can see it in people who can't be with pain because they have a lot of it inside themselves. I can see that was me in the past.

Another positive thing about my illness was that I walked into a world I couldn't ever quite reach before. It's hard to explain but there was this longing in me for years to be living in a different way but I couldn't ever quite get there. When I was really busy living in the city I used to go up to this place in the mountains on the weekends and I would always feel this sadness in me, a longing for something that the mountains embodied. I think now that what they embodied was 'being'. It felt like things just *were* and I think I *wasn't*. I was really struggling with trying to prove who I was, trying to earn my place in the world, to earn my value.

I used to feel that longing and now here I am! I'm here. I don't think I would have had the courage to just say, 'I'm going to leave my job and go and live a quiet life and maybe consider other things I might be. I didn't have the resources to get me there, neither the consciousness nor the conviction, before this.

Illness has got you there.

Yes. 'Try another route next time!' But you can't, because it requires a breaking down of yourself, that's why you can't get there any other way, because you have to break. The ego has to crumble, which it did.

What sort of healing practices or techniques have you found useful in your healing?

On the physical level, I've been on Chinese herbs over the last year and a half and I have had a dramatic improvement in my health. That was almost immediate and then it just kept getting better. I did acupuncture as well, which was helpful for a while. The therapy I did with the yoga therapist/Ayurvedic doctor, which was a mixture of things, certainly informed by psychotherapy and Tantric yogic philosophy, was invaluable. Even though I was really sick while I was seeing him and didn't feel I was getting physically better from the work we did, I see now how these sessions provided an anchor for a deep process of healing. They offered a framework for understanding or coming to terms with what was happening, and trying to just be with it, and that was profound. I saw him for about two years and what I gained from that experience was just incredible. What an incredible thing to have had the opportunity to do in a way.

I think the philosophy has helped me. You need to find meaning in such a difficult experience. It doesn't mean you need to impose a meaning or adopt a viewpoint, but you need to know for yourself what's going on. I think that is one of the biggest struggles with illness. I think I am coming to an understanding through Ayurveda and yoga.

I know I got to a point of despair when I was living in a hut for a while in the mountains. I was really sick and I couldn't go to the house to get any food. I was just lying there and I remember thinking, 'Well, there's not much point in this is there? This isn't a life; this is just an existence. I'm just lying here.' It was really confronting. I told that to my doctor. I said, 'I think I've actually lost what the purpose is.' He said, 'Your purpose is to connect to every moment.' That was so profound; it just shifted me around because it meant I had to connect to that moment as well. I had just wanted to connect to the good moments. It sounds simple now but I just knew when he said it that that was the purpose, I knew that I had to engage with what was happening and not push it away any more.

> 'Before, when I saw people's pain, I wanted to save them, but when I got close to their pain I felt confronted, almost repulsed by it.'

From then on I made some dramatic life changes. I made some decisions, for example I decided to consider a day as half a day. If I was up for a couple of hours in the morning then the afternoon had to be spent completely in rest, sometimes with my eyes blacked out, in bed. If I decided I only had half a day then it didn't feel that I was losing the day. I made a whole lot of decisions like that. I made some really strict rules and that's when I started getting better. Resting fully. I hadn't really allowed myself to rest, I was just too anxious about what was happening.

Were there any particular things that you did, like practices?

With my doctor's guidance I ditched the yoga practice I was doing and started doing breathing practices. I see illness as happening on so many levels; what I kept coming to was this really deep anxiety. I'm not saying it's the cause of the illness but I kept feeling that for me it was a really core thing. So I did lying down breathing practices and meditation, as often I couldn't sit because my muscles were too sore. These practices were really helpful in trying to relax deeply. I don't feel I knew how to deeply relax and I think that's again what was causing the illness. I just didn't know how to relax. I was doing yoga but I wasn't doing it properly. It's only in the last couple of years that I've been able to sit and return to my sitting practice, which is a bit of an anchor for me. I couldn't do that before.

There was lots of frustration and judgement within me: 'If you can't sit and meditate, then maybe it's a spiritual problem and you're not far on the path.' And people would say things like that to me as well, which only encouraged this inner judgement. People would say, 'It's a spiritual block.' And although I'd think, 'That's just crap,' part of me actually believed it because I didn't know what was going on. You wonder, 'Am I resisting?' There would be all this turmoil: 'Am I creating this illness? Do I not want to get better enough?' All that struggle.

Fuel to give yourself a hard time?

Yes, lots of judgement. I think it's out there and if you've got judgement within you, you just pick up on it. It's really dangerous. I think yoga has been the core of my practice. Learning to try to be in the moment, whatever that moment brings. That's the basis of it. I've written a lot, I guess it's something I always do; it helps sometimes to articulate stuff. I keep a journal as well as write articles about the process of what I've gone through. It's helpful. I was given specific *pranayama* [yogic breathing] practices, things that would build strength. I started to understand how to improve my *agni* [digestive capacity] and to understand the *chakras* [psychic centres in the subtle body] and which ones to focus on, using visualisation and psychic awareness to develop strength in that psychic way.

The next thing I wanted to ask was, where do you draw your strength from?

Actually, initially I found my strength through someone else because my doctor was the person who was trying to get me to know that it was there. But I didn't feel it was there because when your body is debilitated you identify with your body and you think, 'All I can feel is weakness. I can't find my strength any more. I've lost my strength.'

So I think through meditation practice and the teachings of Vedanta, which teaches 'I am not the body', I was able to see that I'm not just my illness. It was such a liberating thought, thinking I'm not my body, because it meant that I am something beyond that – that this illness is actually in me, but is not me. I came to see my illness as my teacher, a hard teacher; a really hard teacher. But I see it as the teacher who is within me and I have to honour and respect my teacher, if I'm to learn.

That's not being kicked down by the teacher, it's just really developing relationship with the teacher. I think what it is too, is to develop relationship with yourself. Then you learn to really honour the symptoms, honour the body and listen to it because it's the one that knows. But at first you think your body is against you. When you're sick you think ... I still hear people say it now, people say, 'Oh, this stupid body of mine,' as if, 'I'm okay, it's just this stupid illness or this stupid body.'

You do feel that, you feel so let down by your body. You think, 'I want to do this; I want to be doing that course'. You feel you know at the bottom of your heart that this is what you want to be doing. And your body is just going, 'No way, I can't.' That's really hard; you feel an absolute split within you.

There is that school of thought that says, 'If you follow what you want to be doing you'll do it. If you really want to be well, you'll be well.' But I don't agree.

I think it's much more complex. Really when people are talking about 'you', they are talking about the ego. There's more going on, that's what I've learnt. There's just much more going on. We are just not as in control as much as we think we are or want to be.

I've learned to trust, that's another thing I want to say. Trust is the antidote to fear, isn't it? And fear is part of my nature. So I always know that whenever I go into the fear again I can say, 'Okay, well the antidote I've discovered is trust.' So I have to start working really hard on that one, pedalling fast.

How do you understand the process of healing, given your experience?

I think it's coming into relationship with yourself. I don't think that A plus B equals C. I think people say, when they get better, 'You just have to do this.' I don't agree. As our nature is individual, so is our healing. I think you search for things that resonate deeply with your being and that's why some people heal themselves from cancer and some people can't. People ask, 'Should I do that diet?' But it's not necessarily going to work because it's a question of resonance. So I think it's coming into a relationship with who you really are rather than who you think you should be or who other people think you should be.

Anna's story

In 1981, at the age of 24 and not long after completing a stressful first year as a secondary school teacher, Anna had a psychotic episode. Over a period of several months she lost touch with everyday reality as we know it, to the extent that she believed the Third World War had started between the Christians and the Buddhists. Her psychotic episode was triggered by 'magic' mushrooms and her regular use of marijuana. A couple of months into her breakdown, at her parents' insistence, Anna was admitted to a private hospital and treated with anti-psychotic drugs. After three weeks in hospital Anna emerged fragile and fragmented, her life changed forever.

Her first blessing was the spark of insight upon leaving hospital that there was a problem. Despite the seductive quality of some aspects of the reality she had experienced, she knew in some way that her mind had been led astray. Without this initial understanding Anna feels sure that no journey could have been made. From that point on she commenced a slow and arduous healing journey lasting almost a decade while she struggled to repair the rent in the fabric of her mind.

I first met Anna at a Buddhist meditation retreat centre in the Blue Mountains outside of Sydney. On the tenth and final day of the silent retreat participants are allowed to speak, and not surprisingly most of the meditators start chattering like monkeys after the rigours of enforced silence. It was at this time that our friendship was formed and it has been one that I have drawn a lot of strength from over the years. Not long after this retreat Anna told me of her psychotic episode and subsequent experience, which I found intriguing because at that time I was in training to become a psychiatrist. When the idea for this book first came into my mind, I naturally thought of Anna and her remarkable story. At present Anna teaches music to children and lives with a friend in rural New South Wales. The dark days of her psychotic episode are very much in the past.

Anna, how long would you say you were actually psychotic?

About three to four months. If I'd had episodes before or I had had people around me who recognised psychosis I would have gone into hospital about three months before I eventually did. And I say that with the experience of having a close relative who at that point when I got ill had never had any mental illness. But since then I've had a lot of experience with this person and can recognise the very first signs of someone going psychotic and losing touch with what we call reality, which is reality in the common usage of the word.

So how did you progress after your release from hospital? What happened then?

I had to have somebody looking after me. I couldn't drive. Mentally, I really identified with feeling like I was about eight or nine years old. I hated it. By the time I left hospital I realised there was a problem. I felt that despite all the paranoia, I'd been glimpsing truths about life, about the spiritual world, that ordinarily I didn't glimpse. So to me the whole experience had been really rather special, but I realised there must be a problem. I hadn't really grasped the truth of my situation. Before this episode I'd been a fairly independent person, I mean I'd been able to hop in the car and just drive off wherever I wanted to. But after leaving hospital I couldn't even drive a car.

It was too scary for you?

It was too scary. It was like I didn't know what to do any more. I felt like I was about eight and hadn't actually learnt to drive. So I thought there's got to be something wrong if I can't drive and they've had to put me into hospital. I felt if my parents are having to look after me I must have missed something. There was this knowledge that crept through into my brain: 'There's something wrong.' I thought I'd grasped the 'Truth' but I must have missed something. I didn't really grasp it or I only grasped 'partial Truth' because otherwise this lack of independence wouldn't be happening. So I was aware that there was a major problem on my hands [chuckling] and the problem was with *me*. I understood that my parents were going to look after me and I was still on this medication, which I hated being on. I don't quite know why. I was very agitated, that must have been one of the side effects of the drugs that I was on. I don't even know what it was that I was on. But I couldn't stop my muscles from moving around and I had to keep walking all over the place. I think I just got fed up with those tablets and stopped taking them after a few weeks.

For the next couple of years I lived a lot in my head. I remember people asking me what I did and I can remember thinking, 'That's so stupid! What do they think I do? I breathe and I eat and I drink water and I walk. What a ridiculous question to ask!' I've got a fair few blanks from that period of time. I don't know how long it was. I just sort of drifted along financially; I think I was on the dole or a sickness benefit.

I spent a few months with a friend who was an acupuncture student in Darlinghurst because I had a problem being at my parents' place. I felt uncomfortable. I can remember him taking me to see the people at the Paddington Healing Centre and they were really lovely to me. I started talking to one of the guys there and told him about some of the experiences that I'd had and he said to me, 'And when did you realise that those things were hallucinations?' And I thought, 'Oh, were they hallucinations?' And I said, 'Oh, I don't know.' But that gave the clue that some of these things that I thought were going on might have been hallucinations. So I just took it in and thought, 'Oh, that's interesting'. It was like little bits of information kept getting through …

> 'I remember people asking me what I did. I thought, "What do they think I do? I breathe and I eat and I drink water and I walk. What a ridiculous question!"'

Piecing it together?

Yes. It must have been three or four months after I came out of hospital that I spent a month with this guy in Darlinghurst. My parents knew where I was and were very worried about me. They were worried about me eating and I couldn't understand why they were concerned about that. Of course now I realise that one of the causes of my going psychotic was that I stopped eating and sleeping, and unless you eat and sleep you don't stay well at all. But I didn't understand that at the time.

This guy was great because he took me to see the guy that was running the Paddington Healing Centre, Barry. I can remember him saying to me: 'Would you like a cigarette?' And I replied, 'No, I don't smoke.' Of course, before the psychosis I did smoke cigarettes. Then for the first time I realised, 'Oh, I used to smoke!' So that's how much of a different world I was in.

That's a good way for a person who hasn't had any experience of psychosis to think; imagine going to such a different state of mind that the things that you do every day, like smoking cigarettes, are forgotten! Then months later you realise, 'Oh, that's right, I used to smoke cigarettes!' I was just such a totally different person.

Almost like another life?

Yes, exactly, that's exactly what it's like. It was like a totally different life. And the one word that came to my mind not long afterwards was 'rebirth'. I thought I'd been reborn, with a new life altogether. As in a new life, you feel very much like a fledgling, like a brand new sort of person, floundering around like a foal not knowing what's going on. But you're actually in your twenties.

When Barry asked me about the cigarette I said, 'No, I used to smoke, that's right. I wonder why I don't any more.' And he said, 'You really seem like you're about eight or nine.' Then he said, 'How old are you?' And I remember thinking, 'God, how old am I?' I couldn't remember. So he told me how old I was: I was twenty-four. Then he said: 'That's alright. You have gone back and you're growing up again. But it won't take as long this time.'

He explained it to me that way and that was so reassuring. It was extremely reassuring for someone to connect on that weird level and to be able to say that to me. Also he said to me, 'You've just got that child energy. You're like a child in love with the universe. That's what you're like,' he said. 'That's what I get from you.' I think he was quite into, not exactly channelling, but he was into trying to feel the energy of a person and give them a little bit of feedback about where he felt they were at.

The acupuncture student also took me to see David Tai, who was his teacher. I'll never forget David Tai. He was just beautiful to me because he could treat me but I didn't have to tell him anything. He just felt all my pulses and left the room. This guy who was helping me out, who was his student, said to him, 'She's confused.' 'Oh, confused,' David would say, 'very good.' That's all he had to be told. When I would see a psychiatrist or a counsellor they would ask me a lot of questions, it was awful. I couldn't cope with that. It was just very confusing and upsetting and at the time my brain wasn't working properly so it was pointless. Whereas with this kind of treatment someone just felt my pulses and then nodded his head calmly and said, 'Oh, yes, we can treat this.'

He treated me every single day for a month. I went in to see him and he said, 'Bring her every day and I'll give her needles.' You don't often give people needles every day for acupuncture. I think he is just fantastic at what he does, David Tai. But the release and somehow the help that I got from it was so important and profound that I just loved those needles. It's a weird thing to say because they're not very pleasant. Even at that time I used to think, 'Oh, I love these needles!' and I would just lie there. He gave me acupuncture every day for about a month. He came in each day and felt my pulses and balanced me. I think I was really very fortunate to have that. I don't remember feeling suddenly heaps better but I do remember that it was really great and that I enjoyed going to see him.

After that period I must have moved back to my parents' place, I don't know quite what happened. At some stage within that next year I moved back down the coast for a while. I was still pretty fragile. I couldn't work but by this time I could drive. During those next years I did a number of different things. I took up t'ai chi, so I entered a phase where as well as walking and eating and breathing and drinking water I did t'ai chi and that was lovely. That was really nice. I can remember I learnt t'ai chi from a guy called Tennyson Yiu. I went once a week for about six months. I can remember Tennyson talking about the Chinese sages and saying they would meditate and do their t'ai chi and this word 'meditating' came up. And I thought, 'Oh, yes, he seems to know what's going on. This meditating business, if it was good enough for the ancient sages and I'm doing my t'ai chi, perhaps this would be the go for me.' So that little seed was planted that this meditating was a good thing.

I took spinning up during that period of time. I don't know why. My parents asked me why.

Spinning wool?

Yes, spinning wool. They all seemed to ask me why I was doing it and I just thought it was the obvious thing to do. I don't know why.

[In 1983 Anna decided to learn how to meditate and was referred by her t'ai chi teacher to a Vipassana meditation centre. Over the next decade this Buddhist meditation practice would become an essential part of her healing, giving her greater clarity of mind and helping her overcome a longstanding difficulty in sleeping. Anna also started to keep a daily journal and found that if she could articulate a problem or situation that she found herself in and write it down on paper this would invariably help her to solve it.]

I went to a herbalist and I still must have been feeling pretty spun out. I'd done a bit of reading by this time and I'd come across schizophrenia and recognised that a lot of the symptoms described in these books were what I'd experienced. So nobody ever labelled me a schizophrenic and I was loathe to label myself. I was aware enough to realise that, 'God, this is what I went through. These are the same symptoms that I had.' So I realised that there was still this problem sitting there, though less acute and I was getting on with my life.

So I said to the secretary to the herbalist, 'Oh, I've had problems and it's like schizophrenia.' And she knew of a Dr Samra and said, 'He's doing some work with people [with schizophrenia] using diet. Go to see him.' So I did. I had a glucose tolerance test and it was found that I had low blood sugar levels, so he recommended that I eat every two to three hours and go off sugar, which helped me a lot. I've done that ever since. It really helped to level out my moods and energy because often I would just start crying for nothing and it would be related to my moods and energy levels.

It was very difficult when you start feeling upset or depressed or angry and most people think, 'Oh, something's made me feel this way.' It's not necessarily the case, it may be that your body is just not being fed properly, it's lacking fuel and it's just decided it's exhausted. I know that a lot of people go through all these kind of problems; they haven't necessarily had a major psychotic episode or mental illness, but they still can experience mild forms of depression or anxiety. So that was very helpful and I've stayed away from sugar ever since really.

I used to forget to eat food. During that year of teaching when I was living on the South Coast, I used to go all day without eating. I was racing around the place just living on coffee and cigarettes and then smoking a lot of marijuana. I drained myself physically that year. I got quite a few viral infections that year, too, including viral encephalitis. I'm actually quite a hardy sort of person. When I was growing up I never suffered much from viruses or infectious illnesses. I still think of myself as having a very strong constitution and I think I'd pushed it to the limit that year by not eating properly and getting into the habit of smoking marijuana, drinking more alcohol than I'd ever drunk in my life and stressing about work. I'd just burnt the candle at both ends and really wore myself out. So I guess I was a real candidate for having a major kind of breakdown situation, without ever realising it. When you're a teenager or in your twenties you hear older people saying, 'You must eat properly and sleep properly.' But when you're young and healthy and vital and life's exciting and there's good bands playing and there's good marijuana to be smoked you just go for it. Who needs to stop and eat and be sensible?

'Nobody ever labelled me a schizophrenic and I was loath to label myself.'

It was six years before I started meditating at home. I was still too agitated, too unsettled to be able to meditate at home. It was something I wanted to do but I wasn't prepared to force myself. I just felt that it would fall into place when it was meant to. That's the way, ever since I had my breakdown, that I like to do things. I've tried to treat myself with enough respect to know that the organism itself knows when it's ready for certain things. I feel we are organic beings; it's certainly worked for me. I'm not one of these people that can easily superimpose rules and regulations upon myself.

Just allowing that process to unfold in its own time?

Yes, and when doing a technique like Vipassana, that's how I understand it works. I've proved that to myself. On the other hand, if someone was fortunate enough to learn Vipassana meditation, I would encourage them (again with the wisdom of hindsight) to start meditating regularly at home as soon as possible.

So you've been telling me about that process of integration, knowing that you'd seen glimpses of the truth but that it wasn't the whole truth; that there was a problem. Then gradually over time, through different experiences and practices, you were moving towards integrating these insights ... and I was just wondering how that process continued after you started meditating regularly?

It was something that really happened on an unconscious level I think. Consciously I knew that's where I was heading, that's what I wanted to do. At first, instead of having to sit and think all the time and try and work out what happened and why did that happen then and what was really happening when I thought such and such was happening. Later I was more able to just live my life and not be so concerned with things. As soon as there was no big problem being posed and I didn't have to put energy into thinking about what went on then I could just be relaxed about the here and now. I think that was the sign that the integration had taken place.

At the time I got on quite well with my parents but in other ways I felt that I had all these problems within me as far as relating with them. I felt that I had to heal this relationship between my parents and myself. It seemed like such a big thing at the time. I thought, 'Oh, well, it will take my whole life. This is probably my life's purpose.' [chuckling] After a few years I started feeling really comfortable with them and thinking there's no problem here at all. They're friends.

Then I started feeling a bit scared. I thought, 'I'm going to die now.' That was my life's purpose and it has already been achieved. I felt until I could heal the relationships with my family members I couldn't really move on in my life and have a proper life. A healed life. So that was scary for a little while and then I realised with delight that actually that wasn't my life's purpose, that was just an immediate goal. After a couple of years that had happened ...

Been realised.

Yes, it had been realised. So that was an interesting one. Once the experience is integrated, it means that you don't have to think about it any more. It's history; it's fallen into place. What you're involved with now is today. But you've got a lot of experience, like everybody does, experience that you can draw on.

I used to have another way of understanding what had happened to me. It was like I had opened Pandora's box. I used to think that inside of all of us is that mythological Pandora's box and that we're not really meant to have a look in there because it's really pretty damn scary. I thought that in my ignorance or innocence and my desire for truth, which was in operation when I took those mushrooms, that I had opened Pandora's box. And I wasn't properly prepared for what was in there and I didn't understand what I was doing.

But I've been really, really fortunate because I managed to survive it and I've managed to come through it. My life is way richer for it. I would not have forgone the experience, but it took a good few years before I could say that; because it was so heavy at the time and it was so precarious, it was such a precarious kind of journey.

> 'It was like I had opened Pandora's box – a place inside all of us that we're not meant to look in because it's pretty damn scary.'

In terms of getting to the place where you look back on your experiences as being part of the unfolding process, as being history: how long after the initial episode did that happen?

That was about six years afterwards. When I met you I can remember I was just at the point. Before then I never spoke about it to anybody and it was still too scary and I couldn't talk to people very easily at all, about anything. So it took six years before I could speak about it and I remember when I met you, you were one of the first people. When you said that you had worked in the field of holistic psychiatry I felt quite excited and I just had this feeling, 'Oh, this person's going to understand a little bit about where I've been. He's not going to judge me, he's going to find it interesting.' That's the feeling I got from you, which is really lovely because you were one of the first people that I could talk to.

I'd reached that point of healing where I felt that in order for anyone to know me, I had to say, 'Look, I'm just not an ordinary person, I've had this thing happen. But it's alright. It's okay.' That's the point I had reached when I met you, I felt that unless I could tell the person then I wouldn't be being quite honest with them. I'd be pretending that I was just a normal person and I wasn't really a normal person. I don't know whether it was a dark secret or ... but there was a little bit of excitement to think I had had this big thing happen in my life. And it was such a defining thing in my life. It was as though before it had happened I'd been asleep. When I talk about it being a rebirth, I mean rebirth with a capital 'R'. It was as if a huge blanket had been taken away from my eyes. It was as if you have Pandora's box sitting in front of you and you say, 'Well, this is reality as it seems. Now let's open the box, let all these things out. Now this is really what's there.'

You say it well.

So for me there's before that experience and after that experience. Before that experience it was like I was asleep and after that experience, that's when I was woken up. Rudely woken up. It becomes different when I look at it from this point in time. The more integrated I become the more easily I can look back and look at the times when I was asleep and still recognise so many wonderful things. I can say, 'Well, you weren't really fully asleep and when you woke up, you weren't fully awake either.' The more integrated you become, the more shades of grey you're able to see, possibly in everybody, in all situations.

So you came to a point where you were able to express and talk to another person or other people about that experience, that dark part of your past ...

Yes.

That's such a wonderful thing because it means you're really starting to accept that part of yourself.

Yes, yes.

And bring it into relationship with another human being.

Yes. Then for a few years, from about six years afterwards to about eight or nine years afterwards, I could only really talk to people when I intuitively felt, 'Yes, I can talk about this to them.' Not that that's what I wanted to talk about all the time, but I felt I wouldn't really be myself unless I let them know there was this important thing that had happened. I started seeing people as being people who were awake and people who were asleep. I suppose that sounds a little black and white but I think that there are people that are more mindful perhaps or ... asleep or awake. Anyway that's just a side issue.

Then I reached a point where it became no longer necessary to do that and I suppose I was further integrated. To the point where I recognised, just naturally, that all human beings have basically got the same things to deal with. Even though we're all so unique and individual, we've all basically got the same kind of feelings and fears and aspirations. I got to the point where I started forgetting about my experience. Then I'd be going through a bit of a hard time with a job or a relationship or something and I'd suddenly think, 'God, this is nothing! Remember where you've come from!' Or my mum would say to me, 'Oh, you shouldn't be feeling depressed! It's a miracle, look at you.' And I would feel awed and humbled.

It really feels like this lifetime has lasted centuries already, because I've gone through so many different head spaces. It's good to remind myself sometimes. I have to remind myself that you can't let yourself become complacent and say, 'Oh, well, I can just sit back and relax because I've done all the hard work in this lifetime.' Life is so full of surprises that you've just got to put your best foot forward and have courage. I think that everyone in their life at some stage reaches their biggest crisis that they have to deal with, and I'm fairly sure that that was mine. I've become so strong now and I wouldn't have been able to if it hadn't been for Vipassana, I know that.

And there were lots of other forces that worked to help, but that was the really huge one. I've got an extremely supportive and wonderful, loving family and that's been just fantastic. That's been so instrumental. I think of my second or third meditation course when I was so untogether that I couldn't get myself ready properly to get there. And my parents said to me: 'We'll take you. Here, we'll help you pack. We've got the four-wheel drive out the front. Come and hop in and we'll take you up there.'

Lovely.

Because they could see how much better I was each time I came back from a meditation course. It had such a profound effect and they knew I wanted to go there and it was something that was helping me. So I've been really lucky. I hear of other people who go and do something that's a bit different like that and all they get from their family is ridicule and suspicion. I wouldn't have been able to do it if I hadn't had that support. So I'm a very blessed, lucky person and continue to be so in so many ways. But I think that that was the biggest fight in my life and it was extended over a number of years. But you never know, I may be wrong. But I can honestly say, and I hope I'm not tempting fate by saying this, touch wood, but I feel there's not jolly well much that can shake my foundations any more. Some people feel that they teeter on the edge of sanity or the edge of the abyss. Well, I dived full in there and I went to the bottom of the abyss. There's no question in my mind. I was completely insane and I didn't just teeter on the edge. I went right over.

And there's no other, to my understanding, there is no other hell you can go to. That's where hell is. And there's no greater abyss than your own personal abyss, that's the worst place you can go. When people are tortured or go through wars or whatever crisis, that's the worst place it can send you to and I've been there.

I'm not saying, 'Oh, I'm so terrific, I came through it.' I acknowledge that I've had spiritual help every inch of the way. I know I've been helped. There's no question in my mind. I've called out to God, to Jesus, to help and they've helped me and held my hand every inch of the way and led me to the people that helped to heal me. So the spiritual help is there, waiting to help you.

The moment you ask ... there's no doubt in my mind. I do know that I've gone through that. It reminds me of those mythological stories of St George and the Dragon. That once you slay the dragon, that once you have fought a particular battle, you're not asked to fight it again. You can't be put back although you might have other kinds of battles to fight. I don't know whether everyone, in every single lifetime, has to face that really enormous battle. I know I must sound a bit melodramatic, but I'm not. If you ask people that knew me and saw me go through it, such as my mother – she's anything but melodramatic, she's very down to earth. But she is the one who'll say, 'You're a miracle. It's a miracle. Look at you!' I work really hard now, I teach and I still see myself growing and getting more confident, getting more together. Just like anyone's life should go really.

> *I wanted to ask you, this is just a general question which you've covered in a lot of ways, but I'll ask it anyway: how do you understand the process of healing, given your experiences?*

Well the phrase 'healing is self-knowledge' pops into my mind. I see healing as being a very multifaceted thing. I had to take into account that I've got a physical level and emotional level, and a spiritual level. What have I left out? Mental level – ooh, that's so Freudian! [chuckling] It doesn't matter on what level you can work. You might be able to work on all of those levels, but each of those levels overlaps and leads into and influences the other levels. So that on whatever level you can work, whatever feels right at the time for you, you work on it knowing that it will help the other areas. There might be some times when you can work on all of those levels or there might be some times when one of those areas is so raw or so wounded that you can't touch it, so you've got to work through one of the other levels. I see healing definitely in those terms.

'There's no question in my mind. I was completely insane, and I didn't just teeter on the edge, I went right over.'

That contemporary terminology that we have, when we talk about treating a person holistically, is very real to me. It's not just a saying, it's extremely real. We definitely have got all those aspects and you heal through all of them or just through one of them. It's definitely a process. I think the level of healing and the speed of healing for each person has to be a unique thing and is directly related to that person's karma, which nobody else can ever know about. Some people can die so easily, so quickly and yet other people can seem to be able to go through these horrendous things. They're just not ready to die and they don't die and they get better.

The other thing about healing is that healing is learning. The journey of healing, if it's a worthwhile and real healing, I think is definitely a journey of learning. It's learning about the world and other people, but it's really learning about yourself.

It's learning about love. I think that the ultimate answer to everything is love really. From my experience, most illness comes about because there's a lack of love on some level for yourself. And again that just sounds like a flippant thing, but it's a very real thing. To be able to really love yourself, warts and all, is a profound thing. It's a very beautiful thing to be able to really accept and love yourself. I think a lot of people realise by now that the old saying, 'love your neighbour as yourself,' which is one of the ideals that we probably all have, isn't possible until you love yourself. So if you're walking around harbouring lack of acceptance, lack of tolerance and hatred, self-hatred, if that's how you love yourself and if you're going to go around laying that on your neighbours, well that's not much chop. But to be able to see all your weaknesses and your vulnerabilities and really love yourself regardless, well they all heal up very, very quickly with love. That's something I've learnt.

And the other thing I know about healing is that there's healing and love all around us. It's just everywhere. It's just this huge river ... just this ocean of it.

> *When you say that love is everywhere, do you mean in the sense that there is that possibility in different situations, whether it be in interactions with people and animals or while sitting somewhere quietly observing nature ... is that how you mean it?*

Well, I hadn't thought of it like that – in a way that's true. What I mean, I suppose it sounds a bit daft, but love is actually in the air. It manifests in everything exactly as you say. I think we've all experienced this at some time. We might get onto a bus and for some reason find ourselves drawn to someone and start talking to them. They may say something to us that either at that time or years later can really help us. It could be just something that they happen to say, or as you say, just looking around ... I know this is the same for a lot of people, you look around and see Creation around you, you see trees and flowers and birds and the sea and the wind and it's just marvellous. It's the product of love. It is just a wonderful loving place. Now whether or not people in Northern Ireland or war-torn Bosnia get struck by the same sense that there is love everywhere, I don't know. I can't say and I don't suppose that concerns me because that's not my experience. I just have to speak from my experience.

I do believe that no matter how awful things may seem, I'm quite sure that that love is almost tangible. I don't know how to describe it, but it is there – not only coming through different people or through the physical surroundings, but it's like it's in the air, it's like a spiritual entity in itself. It's just love. In my life I've experienced that it's as though there are spiritual forces there for you all the time and they are wanting to help you. They're wanting to guide you on but because we have got free choice we have to ask and seek, truly seek, inside ourselves for that help. Before they (I don't know if they've got rules and regulations) are actually allowed to help. It's like we are in charge of our lives.

I'm not saying that everything that happens in our lives happens because we've wanted it to or because we're in charge. I'm not saying that. It's more complicated, with shades of grey, than that. It's as though we're in charge of what direction we go in or what help we receive. We are able to ask for it all the time, any time we want and it's there. Well, that's what I've experienced. It's been so tangible in my life that it's just blown me out time and again. It hasn't just been a flippant, 'Oh, I think I'd like a new dress tomorrow, thank you.' It's not like that, it's not a flippant, 'Oh, spiritual forces, how about you send me something interesting to do tomorrow.' I don't mean like that. I mean when there really is a true need and you recognise that need within yourself, when you've got a true yearning for healing.

Basically I think life for everyone is all about healing, as none of us are born perfect. We were all born so imperfect and with so much to learn, and learning and healing are somehow very much part of the same thing to me. So it's as though it's just everywhere in the air really, in the atmosphere ... it's the ocean, I think, of love which is around us and inside us. So I suppose in the same way as when I was a little girl, and I learnt that God is everywhere, that's exactly what I believe and that's exactly what it's like – that God is love and God is everywhere, very tangibly. It's here in the air and inside our bodies and outside us and just everywhere. It's this wonderful Love that sustains life.

One of the interesting things about my journey is that I've never been much of a reader. When I was at school I liked to go out and experience things for myself rather than read about them. I've read precious little literature to do with either New Age theories or spiritual beliefs or things like that. I think my journey's been more about discovering for myself what is going on or what I want to believe. Maybe that's why my experiences in a way have been so extreme, in order for me to learn from them. I've got some friends that are really big readers. Over the years I might be talking about some spiritual truth that I've arrived at through my experience and they'd say, 'Oh, yes, that's what so-and-so talks about in their book. So-and-so talks about this, so-and-so talks about that.' I think, 'Oh, really, oh, that's great.' Someone else has found the same thing. At the same time, even if you read something it doesn't hit home to you unless you learnt about it in your own life anyway. So I think that's the truth; that is the case.

I've heard this saying, 'The teacher can only teach you something when you've already learnt it.' It's like words can't go in unless you've actually already, within yourself, grasped them. Then the words make sense, otherwise it doesn't make sense so you don't learn it anyway. There's all these dichotomies I suppose but when I talk about love being everywhere, I'm not saying it because it's something I like to believe. I'm not saying it because I've read it. I'm saying it because I've experienced it, and it's blown me out. It continues to blow me out, how amidst all the seemingly harsh things in this life, how incredibly beautiful and kind this world really is. How incredibly kind and wonderful the spiritual forces are. How loving they are. It's amazing!

One of the things that comes to mind is the way I've given up smoking cigarettes just recently. What an incredible little gift it was. The way it happened was so organic. I've wept tears. I think I said to you before, I've wept tears of gratitude. It was just completely taken out of my hands, I was sent this little illness, and everything just fell in.

[Anna came down with pneumonia a few months prior to this interview and had to give up smoking cigarettes at that time. The illness and the necessary period of abstaining from smoking during her treatment became a natural aid that enabled her to finally give up smoking cigarettes, something she had been struggling with for years.]

It just happened in the most beautiful, most natural way and it had been something that had bothered me for such a long time and something that I thought I wasn't going to be able to do. But nonetheless, lots of times I've asked for help with giving up smoking, for spiritual help, and was answered in the most perfect way. It's just been incredible, though I did have to wait a good few years; it wasn't something that just happened. I suppose there's a certain amount of patience that comes into play with healing, a sense of fate and trust.

> 'It continues to blow me out, amidst all the seemingly harsh things in this life, how incredibly beautiful and kind this world really is.'

The other thing about healing is that I don't believe that if someone gets an illness and they die from it that it means they've been a failure in their healing. Not at all; on the contrary. Healing doesn't mean getting a hundred percent better, that's not what healing is about. I've heard of artists who will go through the process of painting a great masterpiece, and once the painting is done, they then destroy it. They'll say, 'The end product wasn't the important thing. It was the process that I went through of painting that painting.'

What I learned and what I went through ... that was the process. I believe it is the same thing with healing. There's all different degrees of healing but I think the ultimate healing state is complete self-acceptance and self-love, and, similarly, complete acceptance and love for others, for all beings. I think, if you've got that feeling on your deathbed then it's just the 'ants' pants'. Do you know what I mean?

Absolutely.

Recently these kids of mine that I teach music to went into an eisteddfod. For a lot of them it was their first eisteddfod and you can't tell them before they go that's it's going to be scary. They don't know what their nerves are going to do to them and all that kind of thing. You can see them coming away from the eisteddfod, some of them expecting to get a prize and they don't, others being really surprised because they didn't expect a prize and getting one. All kinds of weird things go wrong, a music stand falling over in the middle of the concert and things like that. You get to the end of it and I say to them, 'We go into these performances thinking we've practised hard, we're really aiming for perfection, we're aiming for a perfect performance but that's not what's it about, even for a professional musician.' I don't believe it's about a perfect performance. It's about a learning experience. 'What am I going to learn? What's going to happen? What surprise is going to get thrown at me? What little lesson does life think I'm ready for? What's going to happen that a few weeks later I'm going to be able to have the best laugh about?' It's just a learning experience.

The other thing that I didn't mention through all of this, it's something that is just a side issue, but the part that humour can play, eventually, along the way of the healing process. When a person can get to a point where they can laugh about aspects of either their illness or their healing process, what a healing thing in itself that is. Being able to see the funny, light-hearted side of situations involved in the healing process. That's so healing, that's so much fun, that's a good one. I've heard of people being healed by laughter alone, practically.

> Yes.

Laughter, and I think being able to have a sense of humour.

> *I was really touched by what you were saying about embracing the journey and not feeling ...*

Not feeling as if you've failed.

> *Yes, that the journey is so much of what it's all about.*

Yes. There's a very strong message that comes through some New Age teachings that we should be in control of what's happening in our lives and that if we think such and such will happen, it will happen. That's very black and white and it's not actually quite true. I feel very sorry and very sad for people who may be lying on their deathbed dying of a cancer and who are carrying with them this feeling that they somehow caused this to happen. That they haven't been strong enough or clever enough or aware enough to stop it from happening, and it's not the case.

We all have to die and in dying we go through a doorway, I believe, into another reality and into another world. We die when we're ready to die. We may die violently, but we have to die of something; I'm not meaning to sound morbid, on the contrary, I mean that's the reality of it. I'm sure there must be people who have tried very hard to work with their healing and they lie on their deathbed thinking: 'I haven't been able to turn this around, I haven't been able to stop myself from dying from this illness.' Carrying with them a sense of failure rather than a sense of that jubilation and a sense of that acceptance and self-love.

> *I think it's such an important message for our times.*

I do too. I would go to the point of saying that illnesses, well, in my experience again, it's all I can speak from, they're a gift. They are a gift because of what they bring with them, the learning that they can bring with them. It might be quick learning, it might be just learning for a couple of weeks, it might be a quick little illness. But usually it's the long-term ones, I think, that carry with them far more learning.

Often it's so hard to see that they're a gift. Usually it's only when you're starting to break through and understand that you are getting some really good learning from it that you start to [see an illness as a gift]. But sometimes right in the midst of a severe stage of an illness you can get this sense of peace and acceptance. I think that they are a gift and it doesn't mean that you're meant to hang on to them. It's like any gift that's given to you. You're meant to open it and use it, and it might break. If it's chocolates or something it will get eaten up. I feel that sometimes we recognise that but we do need to remind ourselves of it sometimes. Because there is also that feeling that unless I'm really healthy and together then I'm not quite worthy and it's not true at all.

> *Yes. So one needs to almost cherish the opportunity that is presenting itself in your life ...*

Yes.

> *To really accept it rather than to ...*
> *[together] ... push it away.*

Yes. It can be really difficult.

Finally, Anna, what advice do you have for others who are facing serious illness?

Go with it; embrace it. Really embrace it. It's an adventure, like most adventures it's going to be really hard at times and really interesting at other times. When you say a 'serious illness' you would imagine that there is a possibility of death with a serious illness and [we need to] understand straightaway, 'Yes, we will all die of something.' That's the harsh reality, that we will all die of something. So it's not really the crux of the matter, and when we do die, it will take care of itself. It's nothing to be too concerned about.

To embrace an illness as one of those things that our life throws at us for really good reasons. It's not just something arbitrary or coincidental or nasty. It is a gift, this is life saying to you, 'This is the best way that we good spiritual forces know to help you learn and grow.' And take courage! And 'seek and you shall find' and all those sorts of things.

Certainly it's a challenge and certainly the instinct of the human being is to get well; to try and get well when they're not well. That's all positive and that's good. There's nothing wrong with that. You don't have to say, 'Oh, well, I'm sick. This is a gift, I've got to just lie here and be sick.' No, I'm not saying that, I'm saying there's going to be a certain battle going on here, and to know that the forces are with you and to reach out. I often still say, 'The "Forces" or "Life" is with you.' You could replace that with the term 'God' or you could say Jesus. It leaves it more open for people to have their own relationship with whatever that really wonderful, good 'essence' is; that essence that is at the bottom, I believe, of all life, which is love.

I believe that a serious illness can put you in touch with that love that is at the core of our being as well as being around us; that's the greatest guiding force in the universe, both on a universal level and personally. I think that maybe that's what illness is about. To really help put us in touch with that divine thing that is within us, that great source of love. The other thing is just to go with the flow and never give up, just don't. You've got to be a warrior. You've got to rest at times and you've got to go with the flow sometimes. You've got to understand when you've had enough, but when you can, you just fight. You don't give up.

Peter's story

In November 1984, when the HIV blood test first became available in Australia, Peter de Reuter discovered that he was HIV positive. He now believes that he contracted the infection three years previously at a time when he had had sexual contact with several men from the United States. This had coincided with a self-destructive period in his life, during his nursing training, in which depression had become a frequent companion.

Predictions for survival by the medical profession kept changing, the initial six months later being modified to three years, five years, eight years and finally admissions that some people might survive for unknown periods of time. Ultimately he chose to ignore all such predictions and to continue to work hard on maintaining his health. Peter has now been HIV positive for 21 years and the current tests of his immune status are on a par with or better than when he was first diagnosed.

Over the years Peter's sense of health and wellbeing has fluctuated a lot, with frequent intestinal problems and diarrhoea, severe tiredness, profuse sweating, liver pains, shortness of breath and weight loss. In 1987 he developed severe diarrhoea, which was eventually diagnosed as an unusual bowel infection seen in immune compromised patients. Several treatments of antibiotics didn't help and his weight dropped to 47 kilograms. At the time he was spending much of the day on the toilet and Peter began to feel that he would die. Fortunately, a combination of naturopathic protocols and antibiotics finally cleared up the condition.

At present Peter runs a highly successful practice in Sydney as a herbalist with a special interest in helping people who are HIV positive or who have AIDS. I met Peter at a time when we were working out of the same healing centre. On hearing of the nature of this book, Peter volunteered to share his story with others.

Peter, what was the nature of your condition and how did it come about?

Well, going back to 1981, I'd had a few pretty disastrous relationships and psychologically I was in a fairly bad space. So it's not surprising that I ended up catching the HIV virus, frankly. At that time HIV was this weird thing that was starting to happen in the States so we knew very little about it. In 1981 on my birthday – which would have been the date that my body mounted an antibody response to the HIV virus and I became HIV antibody positive – I got very, very ill. I also got hepatitis and a few other things at the time so I really had a combination of illnesses. Then in 1984 I was formally diagnosed when the blood test came out and I was told I was HIV positive; that was in the early Eighties. I'm still here.

When you had the blood test in 1984, was that the first time it had become available in Australia?

Yes, it had just come out and I had this vague feeling, a sort of intuitive feeling, 'I wonder if I've got this new thing that's going around?' I thought, 'Well, I might as well have it tested.' But there was part of me saying, 'I wouldn't be surprised if I did get it.' Another part of me was in total denial saying, 'There's no way I could have this thing.' The irony was that I had the test done and they didn't contact me to let me know that I was positive. It was about six months later that a friend of mine was told also, in retrospect, that he was HIV positive.

So you just presumed that as you hadn't heard any result, you were fine?

Yes, that I was negative. That I was fine, because I hadn't heard and I thought, 'This is serious enough, if I was positive they would let me know.' But that was right at the beginning of the epidemic and so little was known about it.

So, what actually happened there? The result had come through ...

And it just lay there in their folder for about six months and then this friend of mine said, 'You had better phone up because it seems that, unless you phone up, you don't get the result.' Then I phoned up and I was told over the phone, 'Oh, you've got this condition – HIV.' Well, actually they said, 'You've got AIDS.' At that time the whole sense of differentiation of AIDS and HIV was not known. So I then asked, 'Well, what do I do? Where am I heading? What time do I have?' And he sort of said, 'Six months,' and then basically hung up on me.

How did that make you feel?

Well, fairly devastated. I mean part of me was totally numb with shock. Part of me was horrified. Another other part of me, it's embarrassing for me to say, another part of me was strangely happy because at that time I was very unhappy. I was in a very destructive state of mind and I really wanted out. But with my philosophical beliefs about karma, reincarnation and so on, there was no way that I could go and blow my brains out. So there was a part of me that was saying, 'Oh, well, I've got my ticket. I don't have to blow my brains out. I'll be gone in six months and then it's all over.' So I had these three primary states of mind and that was very confusing.

> 'I found myself becoming the nurturer for a lot of the people who were freaking out. After a while I couldn't handle that so I basically shut up and didn't share it ….'

Yes, it sounds very confusing ... overwhelming.

Yes, the difficulty then was in trying to share it with friends. Because so little was known about its route of infectivity, my friends were very vulnerable. Some people really freaked out because they felt they could get it from me, like socially. Other friends – I think this is a common thing that happens a lot for people who are diagnosed with cancer or anything else – went to pieces and then needed to be bolstered and strengthened and counselled and supported. When, in fact, the person who has just been given the diagnosis really needs the sustaining at that time. So I found myself becoming the sustainer and the nurturer for a lot of the people who were freaking out. After a while I just couldn't handle that any more so I basically shut up and didn't share it for a while. That was a phase but ...

So you had to become your own counsellor and your own confidante?

Yes, in a sense, and just carry it with you. Because they didn't have the counselling systems that they have now, set up. It was basically that you had the virus and you sort of dealt with it. So much was not known about what you had or what it meant really, etc. Nowadays, if you are diagnosed with it, you have instant counselling support and you've got all these services that you can tap into. I'm really happy to know that that's there. But there's a tiny part of you that feels cheated, not so much now but certainly in the first few years, once those things started to come through. I felt so cheated that I didn't have that support at the time. It's no big deal now.

Peter, could you say a little bit about your experience of illness since 1981?

In 1981 I was very sick and it took me several years to get over it. I had lots of health problems, a lot of lethargy, tiredness, diarrhoea and all sorts of things. Then I found that as I started to instigate a natural therapeutic regime I started to slowly improve. In fact, the longer I survived on one level the better I started to become physically. The allergies got more under control. The concomitant low blood sugar I experienced started to settle down a lot. So the years went by and I started to get better.

When you say a natural therapeutic regime, I'm not quite sure what you mean?

Oh, okay – herbs, vitamins, dietary changes, homeopathy and then later came in things like rebirthing, counselling. What else? Kinesiology, NLP [neurolinguistic programming], hypnotherapy. There is an enormous range of things that this has encouraged me to explore, but basically in those days it would have been herbs, vitamins, dietary changes and homeopathics. That stuff has really had an impact and a lot of it was trial and error because again there was nothing in books to guide you.

The thing that guided me the greatest was the fact that I had the basic naturopathic, philosophical foundation in how we approach illness, which is the concept of the life force. So anything which sustains the life force should also help sustain you with certain illnesses, whatever that label might be – cancer, AIDS, chronic fatigue syndrome. So it was by trial and error, in terms of what could sustain the life force, that I started to learn a lot more about how I could manage this.

And that sense of the life force is something you learnt in your study of naturopathy?

Yes, very much so. I went into practice in 1983, so I was already trained in naturopathic thinking and philosophy and so on; it was very fortuitous that I had that background to fall back on because medicine wasn't really offering anything. That was way before the days of the drug AZT, as little worth as that was in hindsight. But there was literally nothing other than emergency medicine. If you got PCP [*Pneumocystis carinii* pneumonia] they did whatever they could to keep you alive. If you got something else, they did whatever they could to keep you alive in an emergency sense but they really had no prophylaxis, they had no treatment in that early time.

Then in 1987 I got very sick with cryptosporidiosis diarrhoea [an infection of the bowel that resulted from his weakened immune system] and I lost an enormous amount of weight and became very weakened and I basically thought this was it. Nothing I was using was working, nothing the doctors were using was working. We did a combination of one final new antibiotic, I cannot remember what it was, and some other new herbs and it did the trick and I started to pick up again. So 1987 was a very bad time for health. I've certainly had grumbling health issues all along and certain issues have got worse, like gut problems. So that's a bit of a history of how things have gone over the years.

What have you found, in terms of techniques or practices, most useful during this period of illness?

My herbs and vitamins, homeopathics, the tools that I've been trained in, have been some of the most powerful things to keep me alive. And I found that, if I stopped those, then I would inevitably start to go downhill, and often quite powerfully downhill. So those were the things that really sustained me and kept me going.

On a more metaphysical level, counselling has been incredibly important to me. I've had a lot of counselling over the years since the diagnosis, mind you. Sometimes it's a bit hard to tease out just where the need for the counselling came from. A lot of it was just being a therapist in overload with my therapeutic practice and trying to deal with that stuff. Then there were other things that related specifically to my own personal life journey. I guess it's been a curse and a blessing being a therapist and having HIV because in one sense it has forced me to do a lot of experimentation on myself. From these therapeutic experiments I got answers that I could use for my clientele, who were HIV positive at the time. So I've learnt enormously and I think I would never have learnt this much if I had not had this condition myself.

But the curse of it has been being positive and dealing with a lot of HIV clients in all degrees of illness and wellness. It was as if every time I was seeing myself sitting there, particularly with the end-stage patients, so it's a constant confrontation of my own mortality and where I would probably inevitably end up. That has been very confronting at times. I'm not afraid of dying. I mean it's really made me learn to live with my mortality and the fact that death is inevitable for all of us and it's a very natural occurrence in what we call life. I think I've really sorted out a lot of stuff about death. What I'm afraid of is that interim before you die, that phase where you lose your control, where you are dependent on others, where I might possibly have an illness that is very painful or very disfiguring like Kaposi's sarcoma [a form of skin cancer].

The thing that I fear most is dementia. I pride myself on my mind and I depend upon that a lot. Who doesn't? For me it's very important with my writing and my lecturing and so on, so when I get clients in front of me who are demented it's very difficult to cope with, hence the need for counselling in that sense and that's been a powerful tool.

I wanted to ask you, how do you understand why you got sick?

As I mentioned earlier, in the early Eighties I had a lot of issues about self-worth and about self-acceptance, because I was still coming from the era when being gay was not very acceptable at all. That has changed a lot in our community, but in those days to be gay and then to have this God given punishment for being gay! And coming from a Catholic background, which is horrendously masochistic, sadistic, sick and guilt provoking, I really had very little self-substance to keep me going.

There was a lot of lack of integrity about myself in who I was, the value I had as a human being. So I started to become very destructive in my life in the sense that I was using sex as a drug to blot out a lot of my personal pain. In those days, of course, that was encouraged. That was the liberation time within the gay movement; it was the early stage of coming out. One way to prove yourself as being a mature, together, hip person was to be able to notch up on your stick of conquests every night, half a dozen notches. Which in hindsight is absolutely barbarous and very dishonouring of us as human beings. We were treating each other as lumps of meat. Of course there was a lot of fun, there was a lot of pleasure, but also it was a destructive path that a lot of us were on. So it's not surprising that I got HIV. I mean God knows, I had enough sexual contacts to fill a lifetime and a lot of it was very unloving. It was basically very physical stuff and along with my mind-set, HIV, I think, was a natural consequence.

> 'I guess it's been a curse and a blessing being a therapist and having HIV because … it has forced me to do a lot of experimentation on myself.'

So I can understand it and particularly with HIV being seen, at that time, as an inevitable death sentence basically for everybody who got it. Certainly it was, for me, the ticket that I wanted to get off this plane of reality. Because from childhood onward I have had rather severe problems dealing with this reality and accepting the barbarity, the cruelty, the injustice, the whole shemozzle of what life is, and the unfairness of it so often. Not so much in my life, because I think in many ways my life has been a very blessed and very protected life. But certainly seeing the suffering out there and trying to get an esoteric basis to making it acceptable. I still to this day haven't found that. I mean, sure, karma and reincarnation gives you a construct but it still does not give answers for me to some fundamental problems. I did not really want to be here, so God knows HIV was really the perfect way to manifest or create a reality that didn't have to involve sticking my head in an oven or blowing my brains out. So I have to give myself ten out of ten for manifesting a very cleverly devised exit ticket.

Absolutely, you did well! I think you have touched on this, but I will ask it anyway: what have been the most difficult things about being sick?

Other than in 1981 when I was very ill and I thought I might really exit because I felt so ill, and then in 1987 when again I really thought I might leave the planet when I was so ill, other than that, it's just been grumbling chronic things that are not really life threatening. One of the things that has been hard is that every little ache or pain is very easily blown up into, 'Oh, God, this is PCP,' or every little bruise is, 'Shit, Kaposi's sarcoma is starting,' or you get a bit of diarrhoea from eating the wrong thing and you think, 'Oh, God, this is cryptosporidiosis coming back again.' So it's finding the balance where, 'Yes, I've got HIV. I'm alive so I'm going to get colds and flu and that is just part of life.' And just being okay around that. Also keeping really on target so that if it is anything more, I'm on the spot for something to do for it. That is a constant struggle.

I guess you just live every day with your mortality. Even the thought of having an accident and needing an anaesthetic, the hassle that you have to go through medically to explain that you are HIV positive. That is not so much of a problem now because I think medicine has really come to grips with it 95 percent of the time. But in those days it was still rubber gloves and gowns. I mean you really were a leper. So that was very hard to live with, all these potentialities and yet not trying to get too neurotic about it.

The other thing that was very hard to live with was the rejection on the sexual level. These are general comments but I think generally speaking I have had a lot of rejection in meeting someone sexually. Feeling obliged to share with them what my status was, I think is only fair. In fact now that is a legal requirement. Then the look of fear or horror in their face and 'Oh, look, I've just forgot, I've got to meet someone now,' or some sort of obvious excuse to get the hell out of there. You can only take so many rejections before that starts to really affect your self-worth as well. So having to live with the idea that you really are damaged goods and not really acceptable any more, except perhaps to someone else who is also damaged goods.

So it's made me very withdrawn from the gay scene. But that's not the only reason. I have a lot of other issues about the gay scene. But it hasn't helped, to have to go and try and meet someone and then that inevitable, 'Oh, God, I've got to tell them and how are they going to take it?' If I'm feeling vulnerable and needing support it's a very fragile issue to be rejected again. So, that has been very difficult.

Have you had much contact or experience with HIV positive support groups?

Well, a lot of those groups I think are death groups ... basically they just sit around and talk about how terrible, how bad each one is and how terrible life is. They really are death groups, all sitting around just waiting to die and they are dying every moment rather than living every moment as much as they can. So I found, and a lot of my clients found, that it is very depressing to go to these support groups because they are not really supporting you, they are 'downer' groups.

'I've never saved for a house. I've put all my money into travel because that gives me a rich experience.'

In the early, early days I actually set up my own support group for HIV-positive people to meet and to do meditation and to go on bushwalks and things like that, but as my practice started to build I just did not have the time or the energy physically, personally, to organise that. So basically I rely now on friends; you've got your circle of friends who know where you are at and it's not an issue and you don't have to talk about it all the time. That's good.

Again I think you have touched on this, but what have been the most positive aspects of your being sick?

In hindsight now I can definitely say it's been overall, despite the heavy times, a very positive thing to happen to me. It has totally changed my way of life. I've had to face my mortality and come to grips with that. I've had to completely reassess how I live as far as lifestyle is concerned, diet, stress levels, etc. It's forced me on a journey of exploration personally, and for my clients of gaining a lot of knowledge. It has been very useful professionally and has got me to a certain state in the whole situation.

It's helped me to become a stronger person and to prioritise things in life more. I mean there is nothing bad about being rich, having a house, having the right car, wearing the right clothes, but you know in the back of your mind that none of those things can be taken with you. When you go, the only thing that you can take with you, well certainly in my belief system, is the learning experiences that you have had.

So, for instance, I've never saved for a house. I've put all my money into travel because that gives me a rich experience and I usually travel with certain very good friends who allow me to do a lot of metaphysical journeying as well. So I don't think I would have done as much travel if I didn't have this condition.

Are there any particular practices or techniques that you've used in your self-healing?

Well, I've done things like rebirthing and that I found was a useful technique. In the days when I did a lot of it, it helped me really get to deep inner layers of who I was – to understand myself, why I thought in certain ways and why I did certain things. Then out of that state of awareness you can make more powerful or more constructive choices, so that has been very empowering.

I've done meditation on and off but I really haven't had that much success with it. Mind you I did one course of Vipassana meditation, which was a ten-day course, and that certainly opened me up a lot and I learnt a lot out of that. But I have not maintained that either. I'm a lazy slob so I don't do much exercise, so exercise is not a general thing that I have used as a technique.

I think the basic technique has just been to really observe a fairly strict lifestyle as far as diet is concerned, although I can still be found in a pizza parlour or a coffee shop. But generally I've been careful about that. The process that I use is to really set boundaries and as time goes by I'm finding that I have to do that more. So, making sure that I'm in bed at a reasonable hour, then I get more rest. If I don't get my rest, then I'm kaput! I really don't function. So, in a sense, I might call that a process, although it's not one of the usual ones.

I could put it this way, I'm a firm believer in meditation and the value of that, but I think that ultimately meditation has got to be taken into your moment-by-moment daily life. So for me what has happened is that just as a mantra is a focusing point, I try and use 'the moment' that I'm in, in life, to be my mantra; to be my focusing point. As much as I can (and I fail miserably most of the time), I try to be in this moment. What am I feeling? What games am I playing? What patterns am I running off? What sort of destructive things or thoughts am I self-talking? As I'm aware of patterns or ways of thinking then I will make a choice. Okay, forget about that, I'll do it a different way.

So that has become a moment-by-moment, if you like, constant process and that has been for me the most powerful process. To be as much in the witness state of my life as I can be, and from that witness state to be as centred as I can be. Although I lose it most of the time, ask Harry! [laughing] Poor bastard, he catches it most of the time! But I try to be as centred as I can, and to be as aware as I can be of what I'm doing, why I'm doing it and how can I play the game differently.

Where have you gained your strength from?

Friends ... Harry. He's been an incredible calm, steady, strong backdrop for me that I can constantly fall back on. Then, other friends as well.

However, from a different perspective ... I don't know how to quite say it, I'm in a very mixed state about the concept of a God. I feel that through various techniques I have very vaguely touched on an incredible loving energy. From an experiential level I absolutely know that there is a source of love out there. But in my reality on a day-to-day basis, the knowingness that there is this source of love there is nevertheless totally incompatible with the reality of life. I mean the horrible suffering and all the things we touched on before. So I can't say God has been a source of strength. The belief in It has been the constant thorn in my side, which actually makes life harder to deal with. If I didn't believe in a God, in a Loving Source, then it may be easier to make sense of this reality.

Peter, I know from what you have mentioned previously that nature is very powerful for you. Could you say something about that?

If I feel really drained and out of it and needing restoration, if I can get into nature ... I have a favourite little beach that I go to that is just surrounded by beautiful trees and so on. I will just sit on a rock or lean against a tree and just try and melt in with nature. So if you call that God or Source or whatever, it doesn't matter, I find it very rejuvenating.

I guess another source that I go to to find restoration is just a sense of quiet, away from people. I just love being at home with no music on, no television, phone off the hook, knowing that I don't have to speak to anybody and just having time out totally to myself. It gives me a chance to catch up with myself as it were. And nature, in that sense, is a very powerful healer for me. Yes, so that's been good.

How do you understand the process of healing?

I think you first have to differentiate healing from curing because within a medical system those two are totally mixed up or misunderstood. Success is only seen if you can totally cure a person and get them completely out of their symptoms and back to so-called normal. And yes, that is a good thing to strive for and I certainly strive for that in my own life and one day that may or may not happen. But what is much more important for me is how much healing has happened in that journey, dealing with whatever the issue is on the platter. And that may not mean that I get cured. I may die from this condition but that doesn't mean that I have failed.

So healing for me is a process whereby I'm using my condition to grow from unconsciousness levels. It is constantly trying to understand: 'What is it that I'm blocking in my life? What is it that I'm not understanding? What am I resisting in my life?' And that doesn't have to do, per se, with the illness or disease. It's more. I may have symptoms but: 'What is behind those symptoms? What is manifesting those symptoms?' I have a belief system that says we certainly may not entirely create our reality but we certainly have a strong influence in how we manifest our reality. So when I get ill I have to say, 'What is it in me that has catalysed or facilitated these symptoms occurring?' Yes, it may be a bug that I've caught that is creating things on a physical level, but what is the metaphysical level behind it as well?

So that is, for me, the healing journey. It's the constant search for understanding on consciousness levels about who I am and using my condition as the sharpening stone on which to sharpen my knife of consciousness.

And that has been one of the greatest gifts from this condition as well, that the HIV virus has become my guru. And that has been an interesting phenomenon because in the Seventies, all my friends had gurus and I just couldn't find one that I could click with. I always felt left out. And then one day I had the real, 'ah ha!' enlightenment almost of, 'Shit! I've got a guru and that's called the HIV virus. It's my teacher!'

A profound realisation.

Yes, very profound and that created an enormous shift, because from that point on I didn't fight the HIV virus as much. It was, 'Okay, let's just try and coexist here.' And in effect I found with a lot of my clients that the people who fight their condition ... this is a very general statement, because there are some who fight and win, but there are a lot who fight and lose and die. They just tire in the fight. So I try and co-exist with it and use it as a learning opportunity as much as I can.

> 'It's a survivors' syndrome ... there is a degree of burn out, of having to live with this thing and trying to stay in equilibrium with it all the time.'

So your whole attitude to it has softened?

Yes, although I must admit that now [after more than twenty years of having the virus] there is another interesting phase happening where I feel like I'm actually psychologically burning out. It's like living ... I don't want to use the word 'war' because it goes against what I was saying earlier, but it is like being in a constant war zone, constantly having to be alert.

A battleground.

It is a battleground, even though I don't in a sense fight the thing. I am constantly battling life, constantly battling trying to stay well, trying to eat well, trying to think right. I guess it's like going into a monastery and having a very intensive way of living. It almost gets exhausting in the end. You get to a point when you say I've had enough, I'm out of here. I don't want to be part of that game any more or that path any more. The problem is, at least with a monastery you can run away but with this you can't, the only way out is to die.

So I find myself now feeling more and more in a prison with this thing. That although I'm learning a lot and I continue to learn a lot, there's also a part ... I've seen this in my clients, too, who are long-term survivors. We get tired of yet another friend dying, having already had so many friends and people die. It's the cumulative amount of grief, often that hasn't even been shed. You just get numb to all the grieving that you've had to do with all the people that have died.

I think it's a survivors' syndrome. I don't know that you want to label it but it's becoming clearer as the years go by that there is a degree of burn out, of having to live with this thing all the time and trying to stay in equilibrium with it all the time. There are times now where I really get to a point – particularly when I've had a lot of work, and particularly in my style of work, I guess, because there is a constant need for giving all the time – where the bucket is dry and I don't have anything more to give to others. And I really have nothing left for myself either.

And then feeling completely in a bottomless pit, not knowing where to turn to, because friends can only give so much. Lately I've been thinking more, well, I don't know how much longer I can keep up with this. That's not to be dramatic about it, it's no big deal actually on one level, but on another level there is this quiet awareness of, 'I'm running out of steam.'

Physically I have symptoms and health issues that are ongoing, chronic, but not life threatening. It's more a psychological burn out, of living with this thing for so long. I have noticed it with people who have got say multiple sclerosis, who for year after year are dealing with it, even if they are basically stable ... It is all the uncertainties that become almost a destructive burden at a certain point and I don't see any way of getting out of that. You can only counsel so far with it, you can only go to friends for so long about it because they get bored with it too. There's no real answer to it. It's just basically get on with it, get over it, just carry on with living.

What advice do you have to give other people who are facing the prospect of a serious, possibly life-threatening illness?

I think one important thing is you need to become your own authority, because if you are going to depend on one particular system ... and I think the major system in the Western world is the medical system if you are ill. I would say, do not totally and unequivocally put your life into the medical system's hands. As much as I honour the value of the medical system and how they can save life and be of enormous assistance, it is a system that can also be very disempowering and dehumanising and physically very destructive. And even emotionally very destructive because too often the bone is pointed. Certainly in the early days of HIV, the bone was pointed. And trying to overcome that bone-pointing, that death sentence that you are given ... And saying, 'Well, bugger it! No, I'm not going to die for your sake!'

> 'It's a call to a revolution in who you are. And that is challenging, scary and difficult, but it is also unbelievably rewarding.'

So you need to get self-educated, you've got to become self-aware. You've got to open your horizons to a lot more than just the usual information about your illness. Search elsewhere, and you've got to search in sources that are not accepted by the mainstream because it's the frontier research, it's precisely the innovative stuff that you are not going to find in your orthodox official medical journal ... [they are] so conservative, so narrow-minded and ... Anything that has something new or a new way of thinking or dealing with it won't be accepted for another twenty or thirty years, until the old ones die and then the new ones are willing to take on the information. But you may not have twenty or thirty years to wait till you get the blessing from the orthodox system to start something.

So be game to confront your medical authorities, to honour their expertise, to accept their advice but to search deeper. That is one very powerful message and I would say that your life could depend on that. Because if you are just going to accept your chemotherapy and your radiotherapy and your surgery as the only options, as much as they have their role and their place, I'm not denying that, but there is more to it than that. If you just accept that, more likely than not you may not do so well.

The other level is to see your health issue as an opportunity or a curse. You can use your condition to either grow from or to become totally self-absorbed and indulgent. You can become the sick victim and have everybody cater for you, friends and family. Your illness can become a very powerful manipulative stick with which you can really start to control friends, lovers, family, whatever. But usually it ends up in a very destructive way. I can admit to having played that game too at times. But it's not an ultimate path to go down really. It is a very destructive path and it ends usually in your termination, because it depends on you being sick to maintain that stick of manipulation!

So it's using your condition to become more strong, to become more independent, using it as a journey of healing. In the connotations we used earlier, it's a search for meaning personally and at a world level. You need to change entirely how you think of yourself, how you live your life, how you eat, how you sleep, how you entertain. It's a call to a revolution in who you are. And that is challenging, that is scary, that is difficult, but it is also unbelievably rewarding. Don't count how many moments you are really going to have; that's ultimately not the focus. It's what was the *quality* of the moments that you did have.

I think another message would be, don't use every moment to be dying. Use every moment to be living till you need to leave this planet, which will happen to all of us sooner or later. But *live* till you die, rather than have a life of dying until you die. I think that is important.

Kathryn's story

In 1985 Kathryn Skelsey was eighteen years old and in her first year of physiotherapy when her mother noticed an increased roundness of her cheeks. Kathryn was putting on weight and around the same time her periods stopped, so she decided to visit her local general practitioner. Cushing's disease was suspected from the outset; a condition whereby the pituitary gland at the base of the brain secretes a hormone causing the adrenal glands to produce too much of another hormone, cortisol. Cortisol is an important hormone in fat and sugar metabolism and in immune system functioning, and is fundamental in maintaining a healthy body. However, excess cortisol can cause the body tissues to start breaking down.

After various tests Kathryn was treated with neurosurgery in August 1986 to take out the malfunctioning part of the pituitary gland. She chose not to have post-operative radiotherapy. With the reassurances from her neurosurgeon that the operation was a success, she believed that she was cured. Five years later, however, her symptoms returned. She had a second operation on her pituitary gland in May 1992, which again was deemed to be successful. This time her symptoms returned within a year.

Kathryn now decided to find out the reason for her recurring health problems, feeling that there must be a more holistic way to approach her illness. She chose to take an active role in her own healing, declining to have further surgery or a course of radiotherapy. There were no known medications that reliably treated Cushing's disease without significant side effects. Before she had any more therapy she wanted to have a better idea of how to decrease the risk of the disease returning once more. Perhaps in the process she would find a way of controlling the illness.

I first met Kathryn at the holistic medical centre I worked at when she was working there as a remedial massage therapist. She hopes her story of healing might benefit others in a similar predicament.

I wonder if you could say a little bit about the nature of your condition and how it was diagnosed?

In the first couple of years of college, just shortly after I got out of high school, I started to put on a bit of weight. People noticed that I started to get a bit red and round in the face, and made comments about that. I was also a bit flat with my emotions and I lost my periods. Once that started my mother and I thought, 'Ah! Something's happening here!' So Mum took me to the local doctor; he was astute enough to send me off for tests and picked up that I had a problem with my hormones and that I needed to see to a hormone specialist. The specialist diagnosed Cushing's disease. In Cushing's disease, the body is producing too much cortisol. With further testing by MRI and CAT scans they picked up that I had a tumour on the pituitary gland.

So that tumour was producing extra hormones?

Yes, an excess of ACTH [adrenocorticotropic hormone] and cortisol. But I haven't had a problem with most of my other hormones. Sometimes, if a lot of the gland has been cut away, people can lose their other pituitary hormones after surgery. I've been lucky in that mine have always been pretty normal before and after the surgeries. Although at the moment my thyroid-stimulating hormone is below the normal range. And I just wonder if that's got a little bit to do with the tumour and it hasn't really been followed up properly; I've always been a bit slow and meticulous with the way that I do things, and as a result I really don't have enough time to do things, so I wear myself out in the process and therefore produce too much cortisol to try and cope with the situation. Perhaps that contributed to the tumour.

I've had two lots of surgery to remove the tumour, both of them trans-sphenoidal hypophysectomies, which involves cutting the skin and gums above the top teeth [under the top lip], going through the middle of the nose to get to the bone at the back of the nose, and through that to the base of the brain where the pituitary sits, and just shelling out the tumour. They virtually have to pull your face right up off the skull to get the instruments to it. Apparently, both times it was quite successful and I had the choice of having radiotherapy. I chose not to because I had the fear of what it would do to the brain. It goes through the brain in thin rays to get to the pituitary. Also, I wasn't keen on the idea that the radiation would also eventually degrade the whole pituitary anyway. Therefore, I'd eventually lose all my other hormones and lose my ability to have kids which was really, really important to me.

At that stage I didn't have a steady partner but I knew that I definitely wanted to be involved in a marriage and having kids. It hasn't happened yet but it's still something that's fairly important. So for that reason I'm resisting the idea of any further surgery, because what's happened since the two lots of surgery is that I've actually had a recurrence of Cushing's disease again. And I'm not so sure that I'm going to be so lucky with keeping all my other hormones the third time around. At the moment I'm attempting to make sure that my health is as good as possible by natural means; looking after myself as much as I can. I'm still learning the process of doing that [smiling] ...

Join the club ... [both laughing]

And realising the fallibility of being human, basically.

You touched on how Cushing's disease has affected you physically; could you say a little more on that and how it has affected you emotionally and mentally?

Well, I'll add a bit more about the physical because that's the most obvious, for example, putting on weight. Basically there's an increase of fat deposits around the body, especially the torso but in the arms or the legs you get wasting of the muscles. So you can potentially look very thick in the body and very thin in the limbs, which is different to usual obesity where you get fat all over. There is an increase in the amount of roundness of the face as well. People who are on cortisone medication for asthma or rheumatoid arthritis or things like that develop the same sort of symptoms. I have very thin skin; I bruise very easily. People keep asking me, 'Oh, you've got bruises on your arm!' and I say, 'Yeah, I just bruise easily.' I never say anything more than that. Not many people know about Cushing's disease and that I've got it.

I've got more hair on my face, which I'm really sensitive about; you get a moustache and hair around the jowls as well. I've got nice little sideburns that I'm trying to disguise by the way I wear my hair at the sides, and by bleaching. Also you lose hair on the top of the head as well. It's much thinner there. I used to have really long hair and it distresses me that I've had to lose that and cut it short to make it look in better condition. Also, you get really tired because of the muscle fatigue or wasting. You just can't get around and do things as easily as you might if you weren't ill. It's very frustrating. At other times you can get very high with the excess cortisol and get a nervous energy especially in the evenings, which is very difficult to settle down, to be able to relax or sleep. And often I'd get so excited about finally having the energy to do things that I'd go flat out and wear myself out again.

So you're wanting to do things?

Wanting to do things, pushing yourself all the time; yes, that's right. Not outright manic, I don't think it's as bad as being manic-depressive but there is an element of it there, and there is a lot of mood swings. I'd have a really lovely day with friends then feel utterly down the next day and I just couldn't lift myself out of it. I don't like the tiredness. When I was working as a physiotherapist in the hospital wards it was quite difficult. I would have to do quite a lot of physical work and would feel quite drained as a result of that. Having to get down and get up again from a squat was a struggle. Or going up and down stairs. I would feel really puffed and think, 'Is this because of the overall illness, or is it that I'm not feeling too well today, or am I getting older, or what is it?'

That uncertainty of the illness is a really difficult factor to deal with, and I think that's got a lot to do with the experience of illness. You just don't know what is right and wrong, and after a while you become so used to this way of being that you're not sure whether you'll ever get out of it. You're not sure how you could really be, but you also have the feeling that this is not me. This is not the way I should be. You don't recognise yourself. You'd like to be how you used to be, you desperately desire it, really grieve for it and that's part of having an illness as well. You have a sense of loss of who you are and it's just a turmoil of emotions, of not knowing and of being really unsure about yourself.

They talk about visualisation, seeing yourself as you would like to be, and I find it really difficult to see myself. 'What do I want to actually achieve here?' Sometimes I look at myself in the mirror and I think, 'Ah, yes, I can just see you again, I can see glimpses, I recognise that person.' But at other times, I look at myself and I just absolutely detest what I see there. It's heavy, it's thick and it's ugly, in comparison to what I'd like to see, which is an enlivened person, wide-eyed, happy, someone who's willing to express and talk and can do all the things that I want to do. It's interesting too, that there is a drive to want to get back to that. That drive is good in that it wants to get you back to where you want to be, but at the same time it's also a very powerful negative thing in that it pushes you too hard, sometimes, to try and achieve things.

> So when you're pushing too hard it doesn't quite work ...

Yes, like 'Maybe I should have acupuncture. I should go and have a massage. I should take all these vitamins and minerals. I should be eating this way. Discipline myself, make sure I'm doing the right things. I should be going to a counsellor to talk about this.'

> All the 'shoulds'...

'You have a sense of loss of who you are; it's just a turmoil of emotions, of not knowing and of being really unsure about yourself as a human being.'

Yes, all the 'shoulds'; relating to my friends better so that I'm getting more social support, doing things that are enjoyable for me. These are all good things in themselves, and they're all aspects of my self-therapy that I'm putting into place to attempt to improve. But you can absolutely wear yourself out concentrating so hard on it and rushing from one thing to the next and trying to earn money to do them all. Buying the vitamins, herbs and minerals is not cheap, seeing practitioners is an expensive exercise, as is having health insurance. I feel as though I should have it but then I wonder if I'm better off without it in the long run when I get tired. I don't know.

> So it's good to have ideas about what you can do to help yourself but not to let them become a taskmaster.

True. It's a difficult balance; the very thing that probably causes the illness in the first place, that inner drive, that perfectionism, also encourages you to want to be well again. You try to improve on yourself with all that. I feel as though, if I could try and get to the very core of me and turn that around and change then I can head back in the opposite direction. That was the feeling that I had the first time that I had the illness, when I was in college. I feel as though the source of that was basically that I had worked myself really hard through high school, the pressures of the HSC [final exams]. Sleep deprivation from studying late. No exercise. Then I went away to a fellowship camp in winter and it was freezing and I got a very bad head cold and I don't think I ever got over it. I think that might have a fair bit to do with it.

They talk about the link between glandular fever and chronic fatigue syndrome. Mine might not be quite as direct as that but I think it wore me down. Then after that I really didn't get the grades that I was getting before. I was doing excellently prior to that. I'd been a strong student but always at the expense of staying up really late and leaving things to the last minute. So at high school I wore myself down and at college I kept doing the same thing, trying to keep up the standards.

Then among all that I was involved in a relationship, and all the adolescent hormonal highs and lows that go on with that. It was an ideal setup for something to bust, basically, and I think that was where the pituitary came in. It had to go into overdrive to cope. I also think there is a familial element to it as well. My family haven't had pituitary problems as such as far as I know, but I'm told some of my relatives had emotional imbalances, and others had diabetes. You wonder if that sets up a scenario for me inheriting something. Perhaps part of me was not quite strong enough and was ready to become a problem.

A weaker link?

Yes, that's right. Generally the body works pretty well, but when it all gets too much then wherever that weak point is, it gives way. Usually you don't know which part will give out, no-one can really predict it, but when it happens the only thing you can do is do your best from there. So when I first got ill I went through the whole rigmarole of deciding what to do. My parents were very supportive at that stage, and continue to be, but eventually as I got older I figured that I had to make my own decisions about my treatment. Initially I was very happy to think that this surgery had succeeded and for five years between the first and second surgery I was fine. I was back to who I was again. Thin face, thinner, my periods returned, I didn't really have a great deal of hair on my face at that stage – it became more of a problem when the illness came back each time.

I think the trigger for my relapse the second time round was another relationship situation. I was travelling a lot to Melbourne to try and maintain the relationship from Sydney and got worn out again. It was not easy at all. I put a lot of effort into it even though I felt unsure about the relationship and not really certain that this was the right person. I wanted to give it the best chance of working but I didn't feel as supported as I would have liked. Although he was a lovely guy there was also my desire for a great deal of perfectionism again; 'I won't get married until I find the one that I want to spend the rest of my life with. I won't get married until I'm happy and I know that this is the pathway that I feel I'm supposed to take.' That's what's been so distressing, because the pathway hasn't been the way I wanted it to be! [laughing gently]. Even though you make all your best decisions, you're still finding that you're not heading the way you wanted to. 'Where did it go, that life that I'd always imagined?' There's been a great deal of frustration [sighs deeply].

'Even though you make all your best decisions, you still find that you're not heading the way you wanted to. "Where did it go, that life I'd always imagined?"'

So I had the second surgery but I never quite came out of it the same way as I did the first time round. I became unwell quite quickly after it when I started another relationship that was even more challenging to me. This is a really sensitive thing for me because this is really core stuff. It is all to do with core beliefs. It's part of the whole story so it can't be avoided, basically, but then it's also something that I'm very sensitive about and find it hard to talk about. It's not an issue for other people but it was a big issue for me, which was that I lost my virginity to a guy that I wasn't married to. I agreed to it when my instincts were saying, 'No. Don't do it!'

The dilemma to me, once I'd done it, was the fact that I felt committed, bound to the act of giving myself to him, but I wasn't sure about our relationship – whether I could continue it forever – because I wasn't sure about him physically, and emotionally we were quite different. I found him fascinating and perplexing at the same time. So all this clashed with my ideal that I would only ever have one 'partner' in my life; if I left this person and went to another it meant I would have given up my core beliefs. I've always been a really spiritual person, a Christian in the Anglican tradition, but it's not necessarily that. It's more just my core belief with God. I believe he wants people to spend their time with one person, that's how we are meant to be rather than spreading our energies around and wearing ourselves out on lots of separate relationships. I believe that sexuality is a really binding, sacred thing. So for me that was really difficult to cope with. In my mind I got really bound to this person who I wasn't sure about, and it got worse and worse and I couldn't get myself out of the relationship because I was so totally emotionally bound to this ideal.

When you say it got worse and worse, do you mean how much you were bound to him or the actual relationship itself?

Well, everything got worse. I felt confused, overwhelmed. The relationship eventually broke down after two or three years. It was on and off again all the time and I got exhausted. I just couldn't maintain it, even though I kept trying to resolve things. I was travelling long distances across Sydney after a full day at work. I wasn't willing to live with him because I wasn't married to him. But I couldn't get myself to marry him because I wasn't sure about him either.

So I was pulling myself in different directions, and also my parents didn't particularly like him. And that was something important to me. I had always imagined a good relationship with them as well as with my partner, so that when we had kids there would be support from the surrounding family. But my relationship with my parents became very secretive as I tried to protect them from this relationship that they didn't approve of. It was all so 'important' and it became more and more 'significant'. It was not possible to downplay anything, it just seemed to get bigger and stronger and harder to get rid of. I put so much effort into trying to make it work. I could fulfil all my beliefs and ideals that 'love would find a way'. All these ideas were going through my head and

I would start writing them down. I wrote all these explanations about how I wanted things to be, like letters to people. When I start writing a lot that's always a signal to me that things are not getting out and being resolved, lots of ruminating. So it just got all really wound up.

A lot of internalising.

Yes, an extreme amount, and it didn't feel as though I could talk to anybody else about it because I didn't feel anybody else would really understand. This was my ideal, this one-partner philosophy. It wasn't necessarily a religious thing. I couldn't talk to people from church because they also didn't accept the relationship terribly well. It became too much of a turmoil and I couldn't sleep. Since breaking up with this guy my bed has been an uncomfortable place to be. And this has gotten mixed up with the fact that I haven't valued sleep at all. I've felt that it's been an impediment to my ability to do anything, that it's a waste of time. I would prefer to be able to sleep only two hours a day and then spend the rest of my time doing things that I really want to do and enjoy. Anyway the bed was something that signified this relationship that was wrong, all the sexual history and remembrance of it. It was just awful. I just felt tense and didn't like having to go to bed and would stay up really late doing other things to avoid it, not consciously thinking these things but I've realised these things afterwards. I've since been training myself to go to bed and get enough sleep. But for a long time I had very broken sleep and would go to bed at twelve and wake up at two or four. I'd get up to do things, go to bed again and then get up in the morning and be working full time.

I'd also started to get involved in other things that I was interested in, because I felt that I needed to do that to help myself cope socially; being in contact with people at a very basic level but also at a functional level. So I got involved in the bulletin committee at the Australian Physiotherapy Association. I put my artistic interests into that. At that time I felt purely socialising was a waste of time, because it was just light-hearted stuff. It was nothing, whereas at least this committee interaction was producing something and being functional. I got involved in the Australian Pituitary Foundation for the same reason, as well as wanting to make contact with other people with Cushing's disease. It's been good to feel I'm working towards helping others with pituitary problems. But I haven't gotten very far with contacting people personally, because there aren't many Cushing's people out there of my own age. I've also resisted it and have been frightened by it because it's a way of confronting the fact that I have an illness and I don't like that very much. The first couple of times that I went to the meetings I felt really nervous, and teary, threatened by the whole idea of it. Also whenever I have blood tests or do anything like that, I just feel really shaken. I don't like working in hospitals. That's been hard because I see all these patients lying in bed and I used to think (before I started to get more energised and able to get around better), 'I'm the one who needs to be in bed, I'm the one who's sick, swap! I can't cope with this! You're draining me with your needs and I don't have anything more to give, I'm sorry.' So that's all been very hard, too.

One of the questions you've got there for us to talk about was, 'What benefits have you received from being unwell?' First time round the illness was good because I learnt what it was like to be a patient and I thought, 'Oh, this is great!' I was really positive about things at that time and I thought, 'Okay, I'll come through this and I'll be fine from there on for the rest of my life.' I thought it was a cure – that's the impression that the doctors give you when they say it was a 'successful operation'. All they mean when they say it was successful is that they got all the tumour, but there's no guarantee of anything else. I felt, being a physiotherapy student at that stage, 'Well, I'm going to understand how it is to be a patient and therefore I'll be more sensitive to my patients and be a good therapist.' Every therapist needs to understand the other side, doctors particularly; not many of them know what it feels like. But when the disease recurred the second time round and third time round it got a little bit tiresome. So it's been difficult to maintain that enthusiasm for being sick.

The only other thing is that after a while you just learn that life is a mixture of both good and bad experiences. It can't be as wonderful as you feel you have been promised. I felt that God had promised me that if I did certain things and was faithful to him in certain ways that I would be promised a worthwhile life; not necessarily an easy life, but a good, enjoyable life.

Satisfying?

Yes, that's right. It's been rather difficult to think that it hasn't been that way. I remember at times getting quite worked up and being very angry at God and rejecting him greatly, feeling very resentful and deciding, 'Well, I'm going to get on with it myself. You haven't helped me out terribly well here! I've tried to listen to you and do everything right and it hasn't worked. So bad luck! I'm just going to go for it myself and do what I feel like I want to do.'

The reason I'm reluctant about having surgery again is because I don't think I'm going to be so lucky third time round. I really fear damaging my brain and damaging my optic nerves, which are very close to that area. My vision is extremely important to me because I'm presently studying for a Bachelor of Fine Arts. Art has always been interesting to me and I would find it very difficult to not be able to see and draw what I see.

> 'I thought it was a cure – that's the impression the doctors give you when they say it was a "successful operation".'

Another thing I found difficult when my illness was more severe was that I hated what I saw, I disliked everybody and I got irritated by them. Everything appeared ugly. My patients were an annoyance, a hindrance. I hated everything (Cushing's disease affects your perception and can cause depression). Now, through searching out people I like and spending time with them, and being with people who respond positively to me, I've been able to come out of that and trust a little bit more. I've occasionally talked with counsellors, not so much to get advice but rather to get the confidence to talk at an intimate level about my experiences, and express and release what I've been feeling.

I've been doing things that I enjoy and one thing that I've really enjoyed doing hugely lately is dancing. I just can't say enough for it; it has really turned around the way that I've felt about myself. When I am dancing I'm feeling my body, I'm enjoying it. I'm touching other people in a pleasant way rather than having to cause pain to them. Quite often, as a physiotherapist, you are causing pain to make a difference. But here it's a pleasant touch, I get an arm around the shoulder or whatever else, and it's nice. Also I'm not being threatened, there is no sexual invasion of me. I'm not expected to perform sexually either. It's been lovely. It's ballroom dancing that I'm doing and it generally satisfies all the ideals of romanticism [laughing together]. It's been ideal. And it's not too hard physically either, but it keeps me moving.

The way I planned my therapy was that I would work from the very basic building blocks of who we are, the core of our physical make-up. There are three parts or stages; food, rest and exercise. I figured that you need to be eating the right stuff, first of all, and you need to have a good digestive system so that what you're taking in is able to work well, as well. The diet I've been eating has been partly an anti-candida diet so that my insides are working well and I try to get as much unprocessed food as possible. So fruit and vegies mainly, raw ideally, and juices. I have cut down on meat and have less sugar, though chocolate was still a bit of a weakness for a while there! [chuckling]. I've cut it out completely now. It was giving me such big mood swings that I just have no motivation to eat it now. I found it difficult to find the right foods to give me energy, those that give you long-term energy (so that then you can exercise) and don't just give you an immediate energy boost. Sometimes I would get halfway through the day at work and I would just feel utterly drained and have to lie down. I would try to be really good with my food but I was also desperate to have something to give me that extra lift. I found that not many things did give me an extra quick lift except for chocolate or really sugary foods and drinks, which are an absolute no-no. They are probably the worst thing you can have in terms of Cushing's disease because I reckon they trigger off this high cortisol level, and I usually drop even worse energy-wise afterwards.

> *Kathryn, you mentioned the diet that you're on, and I was just wondering what are some of the other techniques or healing practices that you've used to facilitate your healing?*

Diet has been the base, and then I've focused on exercise and trying to do that at a level that I was comfortable with. Not going straight into aerobics classes but just walking initially; getting the body moving, getting the circulation flowing through the body. Then gradually working up to swimming or cycling or jogging. Massage can help get that process started, too; moving the cortisol through the system as well, not letting it get clogged and stuck in the body. I think that since I overproduce it, I not only have to reduce the amount I produce, but I also need to remove it, too. So if I'm not eliminating it properly then that's no good.

So you're facilitating elimination from the body?

Yes, that's right, and also making the body stronger and fitter, and I'm balancing that with getting enough rest and sleep. I've kept a daily diary to examine my habits, especially my sleep and eating, so that then I can change them. I've tried to read as much as I can to help me understand what's going on and what I can do for myself, what vitamins and minerals are likely to support my healing. Part of the theory behind the way that I'm working is looking at all the different aspects of the Cushing's syndrome. Trying to correct them in some way by going back to their source at a physiological level. I'm not simply applying a bandage to the symptoms. That will never work because your body will try to compensate and find other ways of expressing its illness.

It's a different approach. I'm trying to work from the outside back in, to reverse the process. Finding out what is causing the problem and then changing the stimulation or input to the symptoms, to make them grow or work better in the opposite direction. For example with my hair, the fact that it's thinning; well, I figure that that's probably because there's a lack of circulation to the scalp. That's probably because of all the stress and tightness of the muscles around that area. So, surely one of the ways that you can correct that is by massaging the scalp and brushing. Lotions and medications won't make that sort of difference on their own. The same with the skin as well – I practise skin brushing and massage to move the circulation through the area and make it healthier. The reason why the skin is not strong is because it's just not getting enough nutrients. It's all really basic stuff but it's the source of the problem. It's really interesting to go back to Ayurvedic or yogic practices. There's really good reasons behind what they advocate, at both a physical and energetic level. So I use things like cleaning out my occasional nose infections (since the scarring from the surgeries) by washing out my nasal passages with salty water from a yogic *neti*-pot [a small pot, usually made of clay]. And many of the yoga practices are said to balance the endocrine system. *Yoga nidra* [a deep relaxation practice] and *pranayama* [a yogic breathing practice] were invaluable in learning body awareness. And I figure that improving the circulation to the head by gentle inversion positions can only be a good thing for improving pituitary health. And there are other ways of improving circulation for healing.

So there's self-massage techniques and things like that?

Yes, even for the face. The roundness of my face is mainly fat, but I also think that part of the reason why my face swells up so much is because it has accumulated fluid because the lymphatics are not so good around the neck, and that's because there's a lot of muscle constriction there as a result of the stress and tension that I build up around it, which is related to the anxiety of Cushing's. So surely if I can massage the neck to move the lymph flow, and stretch the muscles around the neck, I'm actually better off.

And this is combined with the muscle constriction limiting flow away from the face, and also the rise in cortisol in the morning that everyone cyclically gets. So I work around the face and just try to ease it out a bit, and it changes visually very quickly in the morning. When I got Cushing's disease for the third time I decided I had to turn myself around – that's how I describe it. I thought I was heading in the wrong direction with my relationship, everything was going down and deeper and darker and harder and I needed to put on the brakes. Really go, 'Woah!' to the horse that I was riding and rein it in and then start turning it around in the opposite direction. I feel as though I've done the turn around and now I'm heading in the opposite direction. Another way of looking at it is that it's almost like doing surgery on myself at an energetic level, because I'm 'cutting out' all the things that make me unwell.

Definitely part of the healing was working with energy levels [in somatic or body-oriented psychotherapy, it is held that energy can get trapped high up in the body up around the neck and the head]. That's where I often felt it when I got stressed or worried about something. I felt this flushing up around my neck and my face; I would feel very warm there, very red. I'd have a reddish tinge to my cheeks. Often people say, 'Oh, you look so rosy-cheeked and healthy,' [when] actually I don't feel very healthy at all. So part of the process was to bring the energy down to the waist, 'grounding' it there and then even trying to get it down to the feet. For a long time I could only get it down to my chest. It was a real effort for a long time to do that. The energy would be up for too long and I couldn't do anything with it, I didn't know what to do and I'd really have to fight it down. Now I'm okay at it, but sometimes I will get riled by something and the flushed feeling rises again; but I can get it back down quite quickly now.

How do you manage to bring the energy down?

I take slower breaths and concentrate on where my diaphragm is and think about that area. I'm learning more about diaphragmatic breathing all the time, letting go of the anxiety, settling and relaxing. But it's more than just 'relaxing', it's about what you're concentrating on. Instead of being conscious about my face and my eyes and the puffiness that I could feel there, I take the feeling of the warmth down to the belly and let it open up, and I think about my legs too. Noticing the feeling of the clothes on my skin or my moving my feet in my shoes, or having my feet on the ground, sitting with my feet flat on the ground rather than out in front or crossed, so that I'm grounded.

'Another way of looking at it is that it's like doing surgery on myself at an energetic level, because I'm "cutting out" all the things that make me unwell.'

I teach this to my patients. I'm sure that a lot of patients with respiratory problems have this tendency to bring the energy up into the top of their lungs and chests, around their shoulders. They don't know how to ground, so I often teach that to people. And it's interesting that a lot of the health education that's coming through now has got an element of this to it. Whereas before it was 'just take relaxed breaths' or something like that, and not consciously addressing energy changes. I think a lot of other illnesses can be looked at in energy ways as well. It's a simplistic explanation, and it can't explain illness completely, but I'm sure the energy patterns contribute to the whole picture. I'm sure that with Parkinson's disease there's been a lot of holding of the body and rigidity throughout the life, trying to maintain a level of control. It's overdosed the body and therefore the energies become very 'stuck'.

It's habitual.

Yes, that's right. Also with gastric illnesses, I'm sure that a lot of the surgery for these gastric conditions could be decreased if people just learnt how to self-massage their bellies and get their insides working properly. Getting the circulation and peristalsis – wave-like muscle contractions that propel food along the intestine – functioning better, rather than allowing continual tension to catch them in their stomachs. It's very simple stuff. It may not take much for a lot of health problems to be avoided. There's been some good education of people to eat well and exercise, but people usually don't listen because it's very boring to think about that sort of thing.

I listen to other physiotherapists who don't eat terribly well who say, 'Oh, we don't have to worry about that because we are pretty healthy.' And I'm sitting there thinking, 'I've been really unwell at a younger age than you are now. You can break down at any time, you've got to look after yourself now. It's really important to eat well, to make use of the body, the tool that you've been given to be able to do the things in life that you want to do. Otherwise you are going to lose it.' So the energy side of things has been really important to me, and being able to work on my health.

Where do you get your strength from?

I'm not absolutely sure, but whenever I get to a low point I notice the warning signs. I'm working on getting better at recognising them earlier while they are still not too potent, and they're more reversible, and when I do I always tell myself, 'Okay, well I don't want to be where I used to be. 'So I rally up and say, 'Okay, let's keep going, you've done it before, you can do it again.' It's very much a deep, core inner-self strength. I suppose there's still a self-trust there, even though it's been really knocked around, in terms of my ability to make good decisions. I've made mistakes and I've really loathed some of the mistakes that I've made and really lost trust in my ability to make good decisions. But I still feel as though deep down inside there is this ability and desire to survive at least, if not improve and get better. Although there's the knowledge that I am gradually decaying, as the body does with age, there's still that hope that you can keep improving as well.

Having better health, is that what you mean?

Having better health and also learning about life. My motto has always been 'Life, love and learning'. And 'laughter' can be thrown in there as well. They all go together. Life is about being energetic and enthusiastic, taking opportunities, and it's involved with your relationships with other people, loving other people, loving God, loving yourself, loving your surroundings and nature and everything that's out there, and wanting to learn as a result of it all. I deal with the disappointments by maintaining that 'there is a reason for everything'.

It's a constant process of spiritual, emotional, bodily growth, in amongst whatever is happening. It's a hopefulness. My last partner used to put me down for being hopeful. I'd always be looking forward to things or putting things off a little bit so I could really enjoy it when I got to it. He thought that was silly. It felt very undermining because, for me, I used to enjoy the thought of something coming up.

It also has a little bit to do with my idea of my 'child's eyes'. That's the way I describe that young innocence before you know about all the hurts and damage of the world. Where you can really enjoy what's around you or in front of you right at that very moment and be happy noticing the beauty of things. I used to love looking at things. I've got photos of things, like close-ups that are really colourful, like the intense yellow of corn on the cob. There's no particular reason why anybody else would want to take a photo of that. But I used to love seeing these things and just relishing the vibrancy, the life that I could see in those things. That was where my artistic interest came from, wanting to reproduce those things. When I became unwell I didn't feel as though I wanted to produce anything and I didn't feel as though my artwork would do anything justice because I didn't want to express anything positive. All I had was anger or pain. I didn't want to put that out there and show that to other people, I didn't want to damage other people by having them have to see what was a problem for me. So I avoided drawing or painting. Now, doing the Bachelor of Fine Arts is an attempt to return to where I was before.

Now I am starting to see things again and just enjoy the shape of a little part of something, like the way that things flower or curve and the vibrancy of the colours of things as well. I want to always be able to keep my 'child's eyes'. It comes from an inner source. I don't know exactly how to describe that, some people might describe that as God. 'The kingdom of God is within you,' they say. My understanding of that initially was a very religious way of describing it.

But now I just feel that you do have that glow, that energy, that life-drive inside you as long as you want it to be there. You can die inside if you want to, as well, and be very negative. That's a choice and that's fine in a way. There is positive and there is negative, and in a way I think of God as both positive and negative. There's not necessarily a devil or a demon that is distinct from God. They're actually both wound up in each other; one can't exist without the other.

I think man's difficulty with understanding God and suffering is that he seems to think God is all good. But in fact the whole of the universe is in a constant state of flux between creation and destruction. It exists as a whole entity but it's breaking down and regrowing all the time. I think our bodies have that capability. Although it's degrading, it's also growing. There are also things that you are gaining all the time. Although our bodies may be degrading our life experience, our emotions, our spirituality perhaps are growing.

So the positives of God are inside you as much as all the negative things. We have this amazing capacity to self-destruct and I see all my patients doing that to some extent or another. They are damaging themselves for some reason, subconsciously they are breaking themselves down and making themselves unwell. And that's what I think the essence of ill health is, this desire to self-destruct. And I don't know why. But it's there, it happens. Just as much as everything else, it just is. I used to think, 'Why is it? Why is it?' Perhaps they were trying to get attention or sympathy, perhaps they were trying to remove themselves from a life that had become too hard to handle, and that they had never learnt the life resources to deal with it all. But there are no answers in a way, it's just that that's life; it's good and bad, both.

> *I think you've already touched on this, but I'll ask it anyway: what have you learnt through the experience of illness?*

A little bit more understanding of who I am and how life works. It's been an uncomfortable process of going into really dark spaces and I haven't liked it and would prefer for it not to have happened. I would be very much happier if I could have remained childlike throughout my life, but for some reason I chose to take this path. Though I still haven't understood why I did what I did, I now have more awareness about how my own body works. It's like the elderly who begin to become more aware of their own mortality; illness does the same, it heightens your understanding and consciousness. It's really been an interesting process of knowing how to regulate my body and what to do with it to get it better, which I can pass on to other people.

So how do you understand the process of healing, given your experience?

It needs to be a conscious thing; it doesn't just happen. You've got yourself to a state where you are unwell, and it's very easy to continue in that self-destructive downhill pathway. A lot of people don't know how to put the brakes on. I could potentially have got worse and worse if I really wanted to. I could be hugely overweight, give in to the fatigue and not do any exercise, eat all the wrong things because emotionally they pleased me, smoke and drink to cope with feeling bad about how I am, and basically collapse and blow up and die. I could be a really ugly looking person if I wanted to be. As it is, I certainly haven't put on as much weight or become as debilitated as some Cushing's patients have. I decided that I didn't want to be that way. I had photos of how I used to be and that's what I want to get back to. I may not realistically completely get back there but I will get a better approximation than what I have had.

> 'My motto has always been "Life, love and learning". And "laughter" can be thrown in there as well.'

So healing needs to come from a decision within yourself. I sometimes talk to my patients about it – they might be terminally ill or just very, very sick. Some of them have already begun to give up. Others are not aware how close they are to losing it, and I say to them as I am treating them, 'Look, you've got to do something about this. You can do it if you want to. We are here to help you, but we can't do it all for you.' Some of them feel as though they can't do it and they do give up and it hasn't been long after that they have actually died. Other people have rallied, accepted what we have to offer and come back out of it.

The other thing about healing is that there are no complete cures. I think once the body has been damaged, there will always be that scar. Even with a cut on your skin, there will always be a mark there, it will never be the same again. I think a lot of people think if they go into hospital they will be cured by the surgery that they have and they will be fine at the hands of somebody else's intervention. It doesn't happen that way, and people need to be more emotionally prepared for that. I don't know where it can come from, I don't know how people can be educated in this. There would need to be a whole worldwide change-around of awareness and consciousness of how life works. But people just don't seem to have the intelligence to understand. Sometimes you can only understand it after you've experienced that change in awareness of yourself, and you have that maturity that can come later on in life. That's why they say the thirties or forties are better years because you have gone through various things and you're actually going, 'Oh, that's how it works.' And you have a better ability to self-regulate. And that has all led me to examine the definition of what true 'health' really is. Is it about getting 'cured' by surgery or medications or whatever? Or is it about learning to manage yourself as a total human being, and adapt to the circumstances of life. That seems to be the path I'm on at the moment.

> *What advice would you have for others who are facing the prospect of serious illness?*

Whatever you decide you want to achieve, you can aim for that, you can work towards that. Don't expect absolutely everything to happen right; it's not going to be easy, but if you put the effort into it you can definitely achieve more than what your doctors expect for you. If you do the right things by yourself, educate yourself with what your body needs, and give it the best chance of survival and growth by giving it the right food and the right exercise and the right rest, which I think are the essentials of bodily health, then you'll get through. They will work to support the other therapies you are having.

In terms of spiritual and emotional health, just find the people that are going to support you positively, and stick to them. Reject anything (either inside or outside of you) that is breaking you down and telling you that you can't. Just keep saying to yourself that you can, because you can. You may not be able to do absolutely everything, but certainly you can improve.

It takes a lot of resources to be able to do it. I would love to have a lot more money so that I didn't have to work so hard. I could spend all my time eating the right things and doing the right exercises. But the reality of the situation is that I do have to go to work to earn money to live, so during the time I spend at work I use it to try and keep my body fit. I make use of the walking and lifting as an exercise source, and I eat the right things while I'm there. I try to arrange my time so I eat something regularly, every two hours, to keep my energy steady. I also 'meditate' while I am at work by taking time out to concentrate on my own body between seeing patients or when I'm writing notes. I consciously settle down when I notice I'm getting anxious, and keep myself positive. I concentrate on keeping all those things going throughout the day, not just in the spaces around work. By being consistent, persistent and imaginative in finding new solutions to each problem I face I hope I can gradually improve. And in a way I cherish the opportunity I've had to learn this awareness and creativity. You might want to make excuses for not having the resources or time to do things for yourself, but if you really want to do it you can find ways of applying what you have learnt, even in small ways, regularly. It is a continual lifelong process of learning and applying what you have come to understand.

> 'Is [true health] about getting "cured" by surgery or medications? Or is it about learning to manage yourself as a total human being, and adapt to the circumstances of life?'

Janelle's story

After pursuing a career as an international model based in Europe over almost a decade, Janelle Meisner settled in a small alpine village in the Italian Alps. It was here, while running a chalet and tending to the needs of her infant daughter, that the symptoms of chronic fatigue syndrome started to become evident. With her health declining, Janelle decided to return to her native Australia to seek out further treatment. Soon afterwards, in 1991 when she was 29 years old, Janelle was formally diagnosed with chronic fatigue and post-traumatic stress disorder.

I got to know Janelle while attending an Aboriginal dreaming camp on the South Coast of NSW in 1998 and was impressed by the depth of healing she had been able to achieve in the preceding years. Janelle is a practitioner of Ortho Bionomy, a type of bodywork derived from osteopathy, and a mother to two energetic children.

What was the nature of your condition and how was it diagnosed?

I was diagnosed with chronic fatigue syndrome in 1991, but once I was told what the symptoms were I realised I had had it since 1986. I had glandular fever in 1982. In 1991 post-traumatic stress disorder was also diagnosed. The post-traumatic stress disorder was diagnosed by a psychiatrist and the chronic fatigue syndrome by a general practitioner who uses Chinese medicine.

What were the symptoms you were experiencing?

Well, I couldn't get up any more [gentle laugh]. If I could it would be till 10 a.m. I would have energy from about 6 until 10 in the morning and then I just had to lie down. I literally couldn't do anything. I was also having chronic panic attacks. I was very, very up and down emotionally.

> 'He said, "You don't need acupuncture, you need to tap into the beneficent beings around you." And I said, "Oh, right!"'

So when you said you couldn't get up, you just had no energy?

Yes, I had chronic infections and I felt nauseous and I couldn't get up. I felt heavy and dragged myself around and was short of breath from the exhaustion. If I tried to do anything I would have this adrenaline rush through my body, which would make me throw up. It was a rush of heat with nausea at the same time. If I tried to do anything in what I considered the range of normal activity I would get really physically ill, shaky. I would have to lie down, I would yawn all the time and was teary, exhausted. I would be so exhausted that everything was irritating, then I would conk out. I raised my daughter that year from my bed, she would crawl all over me and I had friends cooking for me.

So the chronic fatigue syndrome was profoundly affecting your life in lots of ways and in 1991 you got back to Australia from Italy and were diagnosed with it and got some help.

The general practitioner who also practised Traditional Chinese Medicine got me to meditate and introduced me to some Buddhist teachers, and that was the starting point. I was also seeing a psychiatrist who did rapid eye movement desensitisation for the post-traumatic stress disorder. I did that for about a year and a half with her and then I went to a somatic psychotherapist [who assesses and restores energy flow through the body].

> *So you started by getting some treatment from a general practitioner who recommended meditation, could you say a bit more about that?*

Yes, I went in every week and we meditated together for an hour. I said to him, 'I would like some acupuncture for stress.' And he said, 'You don't need acupuncture, you need to tap into the beneficent beings around you.' And I said, 'Oh! Right!' Then he said, 'We will meditate and pray and that is what you need to do.' So that's what we did and he suggested seeing someone who could teach me a bit more about what was happening in my body. So I began studying somatic psychotherapy.

> *And that rapid eye movement desensitisation, was that very useful for you?*

That was great. I had been having some very invasive memories and I couldn't cope with them any more, they were in my face all the time. It took two sessions for the first memory to disappear into a thing that I could see but which didn't affect me physically any more. I got a real distance from it, it was like looking at it from far away. It was a really simple thing to do and it was effective. I did it for two or three different things that were invasive. I can think of them all and they just wash away, I don't have any response any more.

> *And when you said before that you were having some panic attacks, were they related to this or were they a separate thing?*

I think they were related to it but they were dealt with at first by the psychiatrist as a separate thing.

> *So you and your daughter were living in the bush outside of Byron Bay and you were getting these treatments and receiving support from friends. What happened then?*

I started to be able to move around and do the odd thing, such as go out to a market or something like that for a little while. I was seeing a somatic psychotherapist. Later I decided to move to Sydney to take the pressure off my friends and dedicate some time to find out what the hell was going on at a deeper level, by exploring with somatic psychotherapy.

I was still having headaches a lot of the time and the occasional panic attack, but my health was more under control. I did have kidney infections and kidney stones when I came down here, but my energy was definitely much better. Everything came out at once!

That's a lot of things to have to deal with. So you moved down to Sydney and started getting some somatic therapy?

I was still very fragile and on the edge all the time. But I could feel the edge. There was an edge rather than just being constant. I could feel, 'Oh, I'm coming up towards an edge again. I have to back off somehow.' Sometimes I wouldn't manage it, but sometimes I would rest in time and I wouldn't get to the place where I would have to lie down. The edge was around energy levels and getting triggered into a bit of madness again.

When you say 'madness' do you mean a panic attack?

Yes, and chronic fatigue syndrome makes you feel confused, searching for words, like living a constant panic attack, my brain felt chaotic. I would have black spots in front of my eyes. I would feel very bizarre a lot of the time. Slowly, through somatic psychotherapy and Ortho Bionomy, I began to have times in between these attacks where I felt more normal and I could notice the 'madness' building up again.

So you had a greater sense of control of what was happening to you.

Definitely, and it was really important to notice there was a lead up to it.

Because then you could do something to perhaps alter what was happening.

Yes, I could go home or not push myself as much. I would be trying to achieve something and would drop it. 'It's not important.' I learnt to let go of having to get anything done. It was more important that I found some equilibrium and stability.

I realised while studying somatic psychotherapy that I didn't understand a lot of things. I had lived my life thinking that it was normal to be cold; it was normal to be in a sweat and cold at the same time. Things like that were just normal to me. It was normal to be 2 stone [13 kilograms] under weight. So through somatics I started to see that people in the world didn't actually think that an easy way to live [laughing awkwardly]. And I learnt there was another model of wellness and life and health that I hadn't really taken in.

It was a real eye-opener, 'People actually move towards wellbeing instead of away from it and embrace feeling pleasure in their bodies.' I didn't have much experience of that, so that was the beginning, that was what intrigued me.

I was learning in somatics to, what they call, self-regulate. I wasn't allowing myself to get tired, I was resting more before I was tired. I learnt a lot from [the innovative and highly regarded teacher of somatic psychotherapy] Julie Henderson's techniques. I was using them all the time and finding they were making a huge difference. These techniques were regulating all the adrenaline in my body.

I was having this incredible exploratory journey inside my body and starting to get this normal feedback, which I had never had from my body. Like, 'Time to go! Or time to stay! Or whatever!' I actually felt those things and I did not have panic attacks. I could feel cold and think, 'Oh, I'd better put a jumper on.' Previously I would just be cold and I wouldn't think there was something you should do about it.

Through the work in somatics and Ortho Bionomy I realised that chronic fatigue syndrome was a lifetime of having nowhere to rest. I didn't have myself to rest into.

What have been the most difficult things about being sick?

Well, the most difficult thing was being a mother and having to raise my daughter from my bed a lot of the time. That was difficult, and it also made me very creative about the things we could do together. What was very difficult was that I had got lots of kudos in my life from being busy, successful and organising things and now I was not able to do really anything at all. That was really hard because you don't know who you are any more, you have no identifying marks. I wasn't identified any more by what I did, so actually I felt I didn't have any identity for quite a while. I thought, at first, being a mother wasn't something that was acceptable as an identity – at least society didn't seem to think so, unfortunately. So that was quite difficult.

Also I got a lot of attitudes from people like, 'You're malingering; get on with it,' that's been the most difficult attitude that I have come up against. 'Push your sleeves up and get on with it,' or 'For God's sake, that is enough now.' That was really difficult because I had no possibility of just getting on with it. I was someone who had always pushed a lot, so if I had been able to I would have. I think that's the reason why I got sick in the first place because I always went beyond my physical limits and my body just wouldn't let me do it any more.

It was an existential crisis, and I was too tired to enjoy being a mother. I was raising my daughter out of a sense of duty and I didn't feel any joy. I just felt an incredible weighty sense of duty to do it well. I did all these activities with her that were the right things to do, but I wasn't enjoying it.

> 'I was too tired to enjoy being a mother. I was raising my daughter out of a sense of duty and I didn't feel any joy.'

Was that because you had so little energy available for yourself?

Yes, loving actually takes a lot of energy and I didn't realise that! [laughs gently] It was really difficult and being with friends was very difficult, relationship in general was very difficult. I had difficulties with people not accepting that I couldn't be like I used to be.

You said before that some people had a sense of you malingering in some way, the implication being that you had some level of psychological control over the whole process. If you just got into the right head space then you would get better. Was that also with your friends as well?

Yes, well-meaning friends and family would tell me to snap out of it: 'You can do it, Janelle!' They would get incredibly irritated, especially women, which was really bizarre; perhaps they felt I was letting down the team or something.

What were the positive things that came out of your experience of illness?

Well, it was like having a very long retreat and I came out knowing much better who I was and what was important, plus who my friends actually were. I had often gone with the flow of whatever was happening around me until that time in my life. I had to really start getting clear, 'What do I want to achieve?' and just do one thing. That was a real will-building exercise for me.

The illness taught me something that I had never learnt, that most people just learn as children; how to goal-set and prioritise. That was very positive.

Lying around noticing the world for a while without actually being able to be involved in it taught me a lot. It piqued my curiosity about other people, I had more curiosity about motivations, my own and other people's. And noticing how much time people spend doing useless things pushed me more and more towards wanting guidance as well. The people around me who I thought were wise actually weren't that wise, they weren't wise enough. So I started looking towards spiritual teachers and that has been very positive.

I got into bodywork as well. I had been doing it before as a hobby. It was the bodywork that finally put the pieces together for me of how to get better. It led to me creating a new career for myself. I saw how it transformed my whole experience of being sick and I realised it was a worthwhile thing to pursue as a career.

Can you say a little about your experience of bodywork?

I tried different types of bodywork and had traumatic experiences each time with massage and chiropractics, energetic healing, all sorts of different things. Then I went to a class with Kath Kain; she was doing a shock and trauma class based on the work of a doctor in the States, Peter Levine. She did a bodywork session on me where she really deeply noticed the tiredness in my cells. She felt it and she said it to me and it was just like this awakening, where I was completely acknowledged. It was an amazing experience. That was a turning point for me. 'Okay, someone can see that this is real, it is actually real.' She made the experience real and affirming, and that was the beginning of getting better.

It sounds like you were met at a very deep level.

Yes. It felt like every part of me was exhausted and sick and she actually knew that. It was a great relief. I guess I was thinking, 'Maybe they're right; maybe I'm actually malingering, maybe I'm actually mad and this is all psychosomatic.' She could actually sense the lack of tone in the muscles, even in my eyes. And it was, of course, the relationship made then that was really important too. She held this space of, 'This is the way you are doing your life right now.' And she was fine with it, she wasn't disillusioned, she wasn't disappointed in me. She just said, 'Oh, so that is how you are doing it, that is how you are living.'

There was no sense of judgement.

No, none at all, and that was so healing.

What sort of practices or healing techniques have you found useful?

Meditation, but little tiny bits of meditation often. Different Buddhist mantras have been helpful. Psychotherapy helped because there is definitely an emotional base to getting chronic fatigue and having post-traumatic stress disorder. So I had to work with all of that, and I had to find a therapy that wasn't cathartic. The therapy I found wasn't agitating the system, it was moving towards peace in the system, it was a completely different way of working than I had ever worked before.

I used to have a lot more energy and I could do those things that they would ask you to do, cathartic processes or long talk sessions, but I didn't have the energy. I found this much more subtle way of working which I almost imposed on my therapist. Then I found that there were people who were already doing it better and I could work with them and I could let go of having to control the therapy.

Julie Henderson's practices were incredibly helpful, jiggling and humming and silly talk and tough talk and all those exercises that are just a vehicle to go back to feeling good and happy, no matter what. My basic practice was, how can I go back to feeling good anyway?

Can you say a bit more about feeling good, what that means?

Feeling good was feeling warm, not shaky, feeling more layers of myself, not feeling like a shadow. Because I often felt like a shadow; a wispy, not quite existing wind [chuckling]. So every time I would get the sense that the wind could blow through me, I'd know, from what my psychiatrist had taught me, that I would have to do something to come back to wellbeing. And wellbeing was much more solid. I would push my back against something solid and feel my spine and get a sense of the heaviness, a weight coming back into my body.

Feeling substantial?

Yes, that's a good word for it. It wasn't about being hysterically happy, it was just being fine with whatever was happening. If I was sad I was substantial in my sadness, but I was with my sadness. And noticing sensation, too; if I was feeling well in myself, I could notice sensations in my body. A lot of the time it was noticing that a situation was too much for me, or that I was tired and needed to rest. So the wellbeing for me was noticing myself more and more; layers of myself inside, outside and the relationship between myself, the environment and other people.

In all different situations that life presents.

Yes, if there were some people over for dinner and I noticed that I had to disappear just to be able to get through dinner. I would get a little wafty and spacey because I was too tired a lot of the time to talk to people. So I would notice that I was not really there and would go into my room and jiggle and hum and lie down. I would realise that it was too much for me. And would tell them, 'I'm not having dinner with you. Carry on without me.' And I would eat dinner on my own.

So, being comfortable with that process of self-regulating and coming back to your own integral sense. Is that what you mean?

Yes, I would begin doing something and then I would have to notice that it wasn't making me feel good. Then I would think: 'What's actually going on for me? What can I do to feel better?'

Yoga was very helpful, too; the Desikachar style of yoga where you stay within your limits and you don't push your body. You did as much as felt good and then you stopped. You never tried to get it right, get it perfect, which is the whole chronic fatigue thing for me.

I had been into eating correctly and I did the macrobiotic trip for a while; all of that went, I had to trust my intuition with everything. 'Does this food actually feel like it's what I want to eat?' It wasn't even about, 'Is it good for me?' But could I be bothered eating it? 'Yes, well I may as well eat that because at least I want it.' It was really interesting having to drop my whole life, let go of everything, let it all drift off. And then pick up pieces of things very sloppily and easily and in a carefree way and try not to take anything back in with the rigidity and the perfection that I tried to do it before.

A more haphazard way of being?

Yes, I could do something intensely and drop it but I couldn't do it in an easy, sloppy way. If I was going to do it, I was going to do it right! [chuckling] That was a whole learning curve. I had also been a very strict vegetarian since I was quite young. That was not working for me physically any more. I was underweight and an Ayurvedic diet really helped. I put some meat back in my diet, chicken and fish, and let go of the fact that I was killing things. Eating what I actually needed. That really helped, loosening up around my diet and finding out what my body needed and eating that rather than having a philosophical diet.

'Feeling good was feeling warm, feeling more layers of myself, not feeling like a shadow. I often felt like a shadow; a wispy, not-quite-existing wind.'

So letting the body speak rather than the head.

Yes. My physical shape changed. I let go of all the really deep muscle contraction I had. For a while I was sloppy and it was so bizarre to look at myself like that. Then this healthy muscle slowly grew back that had its own natural sense of tone.

There was a deep widening relaxation process that happened right from my core and out through all the muscles. It happened in the membranes in my body, it happened everywhere, there was no tension. I had a whiplash neck again for a while when the membranes let go in my body, especially around my head. Slowly I had to get my head back onto my neck and onto my body in a comfortable, easy way instead of a tight way.

I know you've touched on this before, but where have you have gained strength from?

From somatic psychotherapy, Ortho Bionomy and from Ayurveda. Spiritual teachers, like the Tibetans and Aboriginal elders, have given me strength. Also several alternative GPs – one who does homeopathy and the GP who taught me to meditate and pray – and my Buddhist psychiatrist who reintroduced me to my body.

People like that have come out of the woodwork over and over again; very spiritual, caring, nurturing people. A lot of men, I've had a lot of help from very nurturing men. That was a revelation to me, how many gentle, caring men there are in the world.

I gained strength too from joining groups where people had actually been where I had been. That was a big source of strength, seeing there was light at the end of the tunnel and that I would eventually get better.

What sort of support groups were they?

Well, one was a group of people who had chronic fatigue and everyone was using different ways to get better. That was great because I realised there were actual stages of having chronic fatigue. It does seem to have a shelf life of about ten years and I knew where I was on the continuum. I was fairly sure that one way or another I was going to get out the other end within about ten years. So that was a big relief. Hearing other people's experiences of what they had tried, and seeing the very common threads between us of how our lives were before the illness. There was a big 'Aha!' happening. This isn't just a virus. I had a sense of that before, but it really hit me there because we were all such similar people with very similar backgrounds. It was amazing.

What have you learnt through the experience of illness?

I have learnt to use my networking skills to get support and I have learnt that not many people know how to do that. People are very happy to help when you ask them and actually very pleased to be able to help. I have learnt that there is a lot more care out in the community and a hunger for community than I had realised before. I have learnt that I am not an island. It is okay not to cope, rather than, 'You are a fuck-up because you are not coping.' A sense of, 'It's now. Everything is now.' Being more present in myself and being present with the moment: 'In this moment I'm not coping and that is okay. And it will pass.' Much more mindfulness.

Without it being laden with all these voices from the past?

Yes. The judgements of how one should be had to go. Meditating brought that about. It's not there all the time but I am more in the moment than I ever would have been. 'It's Wednesday at 4 o'clock and I'm feeling like shit and that's all.' Too bad if it was all of yesterday as well and it might be all of tomorrow. I had to come back to now. Not project into the future.

Would you say that being sick and having the experience of illness has really accelerated that process of mindfulness?

Yes, I had been toying with it and meditating and doing yoga since I was seventeen and I didn't have a clue, actually. I thought I was doing pretty well [chuckling] until I actually needed to use those things and to really live them. Now that I have energy I can see: 'Wow! There is so much more to being mindful than actually coping with illness.' There's a whole other layer to it now, which is really exciting. I really was using mindfulness as a way of staying sane and now it is not so limited in its scope.

So, given your experiences, how do you understand the process of healing?

For me it's deeply noticing yourself in your body sensations and deeply becoming conversant with yourself. Really noticing who you are and how you move in the world and what that feels like. The process of healing for me is; you come back in and you find yourself and you notice yourself and then you can notice yourself and others and the environment. Then noticing your relationship with God, or whatever you want to call it out there.

In the whole process there is this moment to moment noticing. There is suffering, and finding serenity with that, instead of feeling like you could somehow transcend suffering.

I have realised that there is this coping strategy that comes out of surviving something quite traumatic which is actually health oriented, it is oriented towards affirming life. It's a stress response where you become altruistic a bit. I think something is triggered in people and they start to want to heal and to heal others. I don't know how to explain it, but something triggers it and you get on this journey of, 'How can I be happy and healthy? And how can I take that out into the world?'

That for me is part of the process of healing. There is this turnaround at a certain point where a whole bunch of different positive experiences are let in, and out of it grows this little seed. A sprout of life of health. It isn't just survival, it isn't just getting better; it is actually this new seed that comes out. And that creative force is so important. Once people have got that, there is nothing that is going to stop them. It doesn't matter if it takes them ten or fifteen years, but there is this whole new feeling about their experience. That is healing for me.

So that sense of someone blossoming and that the healing force is alive and well and will reach toward the sun naturally.

Yes, the seed will find its own nourishment and support and a source of joy again. You get your sense of humour back again. For that to happen you have to let go of whatever the story was about why you got sick [laughing heartily]. And that isn't easy! Identifying the story isn't letting go of the story. Finding where the story might be held or trapped in your body isn't letting go of the story either. Every time I would come up against the story at another layer in my body, it was really important to let go again of the story, and just keep healing.

So the story is being fundamentally limiting of healthy self-expression.

Yes, it keeps you away from the healthy self-expression. And people do it differently, identifying themselves as a victim or 'poor me' or something.

Letting go of the story of who I was out in the world, for a lot of people, is very hard to do. I had to find a new identity that included being exhausted all the time. It is amazing what comes out of that, how many different people you are. A much richer tapestry emerges.

What advice would you have for other people facing serious illness?

Well, getting lots of different opinions from different cultural approaches to illness helped me. I started with Western medicine and it was pathologising [viewing physical or mental experiences as expressions of a diseased state] what was happening. Then I noticed that in different cultures they viewed illness with completely different eyes, they did not pathologise as much. With Chinese medicine it was refreshing to think of building more harmony between my organs, rather than thinking my liver function is such and such ... [laughing] It was a more romantic, poetic way of being with the illness. It was also a bigger picture, a wider view, than just, 'Your liver is really sick.'

If you have to go through all the emotional reasons why you might have got sick, it's very important to keep a very positive focus. Go back and notice formative moments of goodness in childhood. I had to notice the good stuff and the yummy stuff and what worked for me and really changed my focus; changed it into a more optimistic, more positive attitude. People get very good at talking about the bad things but they haven't got very good at feeling okay anyway. We've got very clever at pulling all the yukky bits out of the cupboard and forgetting the goodness.

> 'I've had a lot of help from very nurturing men. That was a revelation to me, how many gentle, caring men there are in the world.'

It's a real culture now, isn't it?

Yes, it's dangerous; it's not healthy. My advice if you are in the medical system is, you can feel so out of control while they try this and try that. And then they say, 'Well, we don't really know what to do, so ...' You fear nothing is going to work and you feel completely unsupported. So get as wide a set of resources as you can and get physically resourced too. Whatever it is that makes you feel good, if it is some sort of touch or bodywork or saunas or something to build those resources for yourself. Find places where you can go and feel good or feel as best you can.

Getting into nature and building a relationship with nature has been very good for me. Find support, and if you find it hard to take in support, there are people who can teach you how to do that. You can face the discomfort of having to be supported and in the end get some very pleasant surprises about how much people receive when they are supporting you. There is a whole learning for everyone involved in supporting someone who is ill that is amazing, very healing.

> *So when you said that there are places where you can learn how to be supported, how to allow yourself to be supported, did you mean in terms of the somatic psychotherapy community or ...?*

Yes, that or ... I mean generally there are a lot of different places where you can go and you can meet people; community networks where people have actually been through hell and have learnt how to take in support and how to be supportive. There are little pockets of people doing that all over the place in our society; we tend to gravitate to them only when we are sick or we need help or if there are legal problems or family dysfunction or something. If you go to a group like that or stay with a group of people like that you notice they will share with you all their experiences of being helped. Then you realise, 'I can be helped, too, and it is okay. These people are just normal people like me and they have been helped. They are helping others.

I had such a long time where I just thought: 'Okay, I have to hide away at home and I'm not worthy to be out in society because I can't contribute and I'm ill. I'm boring because I can't laugh and joke and I can't dance at parties, I can't do anything and so I had better just hide and go away.' I slowly got out into a support group or a parenting group and these were places where I could go and talk to people who were struggling along, having a good time sometimes and not such a good time sometimes. There were immense resources of support in those groups of people because they were being up front and real about what was actually happening in their day-to-day lives.

I would say get out into the community as much as you feel is possible with your illness. I couldn't do a lot of it, but the bits that I did meant I then had a whole lot more resources. There would be phone calls or people who would turn up with a meal or something like that, when you needed them.

Really discovering community in the original sense of the word; that it exists and it's alive.

It is so important when you get low and need to rest if you have someone who is willing to be there, take the kids away, cook meals or clean the house. There will come a time then when you are able to give back, too. But the people don't really care if they get anything back, it is a rich experience to do something, give something.

How did you cope financially through the illness?

Well, I didn't cope very well [laughing]. I slowly lost all resources, used up all my savings; I sold the business because I couldn't work in it any more. I sold it at the wrong time, I had to because my health had collapsed and I couldn't do anything. I came back to Australia because I could get on the sole parent's pension out here, whereas in Italy I was struggling along trying to work doing sewing and leatherwork from home. I was trying to do anything that I could possibly do from my bed to keep some money coming in. I thought: 'What am I doing this for? I'm going to go home and get better. I was thinking, 'I'll get over it soon.' So I came home and six months later I wasn't any better, that was a bit of a shock.

'You can face the discomfort of having to be supported and in the end get some very pleasant surprises about how much people receive when they are supporting you.'

I used up every cent I had, but I've had incredible experiences of money pouring in whenever I needed it from very generous friends. A girlfriend of mine sent me $500 for Valentine's Day one year. When I first got back to Australia I needed a car and was offered two cars. A friend approached me and said, 'I don't suppose you want a car, do you?' I had been hitchhiking until then with my daughter and the groceries. My family helped me out over and over again.

It has been amazing. I have experienced so many times the incredible grace of being helped out. Prior to getting sick I had a business that was worth a lot of money, I had money in the bank, a car and a house. I had to walk away from it to get better; I couldn't keep that lifestyle. So I guess in one sense I didn't cope, but if you don't judge it, I am much richer now in every way than I ever was before.

Sara's story

Sara Chesterman was on holidays in Byron Bay in 1995 when she dived off a friend's shoulders while playing in the surf into water that was much shallower than she had realised. The spinal cord in her neck was crushed at the level of lower cervical vertebrae leaving her with quadriplegia. At the time of her accident Sara was 24 years old and in her third year of architecture. After ten months in rehabilitation hospitals, Sara started to pick up the pieces of her former life.

I first heard of Sara's plight through two mutual friends who knew of the book I was writing and who both independently recommended that I include Sara's story. Though still in the early days of her healing, Sara's creative and courageous approach to her condition is awe-inspiring and highlights many important aspects of the healing journey.

Could you tell me about the nature of your disability and how it came about?

The medical diagnosis is quadriplegia at the level of the sixth and seventh cervical vertebrae, which means that I have full function in my body from the neck up and I've got full arm function apart from my fingers (which I can't move at all) and my triceps are weak. Otherwise all my other arm muscles are there and that includes latissimus dorsi, which run down the back.

The swimmers' muscle.

It is! When I'm treading water I get a real sense of that buzzing and my legs flapping around. I can actually move my hips gently with my latissimus dorsi. It's a very bizarre feeling, it's like watching someone levitating a chicken!

So you can actually move your latissimus dorsi and that moves your legs?

Yes, I can see my feet floating and I know I'm doing it but don't know how! [giggling]

Like a whale ...

Like a whale, I love that!

Moving your dorsal fin or back fin and having a whale tail ... You've said a little bit about how your disability has affected you physically; how has it affected you in other ways?

The physical has affected my life in huge ways in terms of physical freedom in being less able to do things spontaneously. That's something that the whole rehabilitation process is about, being able to get as much spontaneity back as possible. That's probably the aim. Emotionally, it's made me feel trapped. Also it makes me feel vulnerable, very vulnerable physically, and that has emotional repercussions.

You feel marginalised. It's a whole new threat to your self-esteem, being in a wheelchair, just going out on the street, watching your impact on people. That can be really difficult at first; it's such a blow to your self-esteem. You are used to being this young girl walking down the street, and people look at you and they think there are young people in the world. They think she looks happy, she's fine. You see that reflected in people's faces.

Then you come on the street and you're this young girl who is hurt and you see it in people's eyes; they just don't want to look. They shut down and you create turmoil and that's a really hard thing to cope with at first. But I think I've learnt to turn it around. I don't know if it's because I'm a Leo or what, but I like to have impact on people; I'm really conscious of my impact on people. When I was able-bodied I used to look at people, it was almost like a challenge, 'Engage with me.' Now I like to look people in the eyes, to take them on and calm them down or say, 'Look, everything is fine.' And so now in a way I'm in a more powerful position to do that because they look at me in shock and in some cases I can make them more comfortable with disability.

I guess you've immediately got their attention.

Yes, exactly. I've spent a lot of time thinking about my character and how I'm actually quite suited to being in a wheelchair! [laughing together] A lot of people aren't and I'm really lucky because I love people. I love having people help me and I love being around people. I also love making connections with people. I did some trance work with this psychologist, he looks for your core values, and I think what we always came up with is movement and making connections. The reason that I'm interested in movement is to make connections with people.

So having a disability is a big blow to your self-esteem. I remember being in hospital and thinking that when I was able-bodied I could feel marginalised at times, but there was always that really strong belief that you can get there if you want to and that had been instilled in me. I was educated at a private school – you are told that you will be 'successful'. So to have that taken away from you, the belief that you can have that money or that glamour or … that's a big blow. Then you lose all sense of yourself as physically attractive, as a sexual being. You know all that Hollywood stuff about sexuality is so much about appearance and physical fitness, looking good, being fit. That's really hard.

I think the effect on my parents is the hardest thing; that's the biggest grief to overcome, coping with the grief of my parents and that burden on me. Because my dad's in hospital at the moment, he just had prostate cancer removed, they cut it all out. I went to see him and I felt physically ill and sick. I realised the real trauma of going to visit someone in hospital, it was so much more traumatic than being in hospital myself. It made me think again about the trauma I put my parents through when I first had the accident.

It was the first time my mother said to me; she actually gave me a hug and said, 'Do you realise how much trauma we went through? It was just so terrible seeing you in traction.'

It was good she was able to say that.

It was huge. It's been really interesting with my sister, because we've become really close since my accident. We had had this whole time apart before my accident, then she flew back from overseas to be with me and she lived in Brisbane for two months while I was in hospital there. Previously I was always the 'good' one and she was always the one with the trouble and being in trouble and suddenly the roles were reversed. We've become really close, as well as her becoming very close to my friends; it's been huge [chuckling softly]. That's been interesting, sister rivalry – who's good at what – that has all come up again.

'I've spent a lot of time thinking about my character and how I'm actually quite suited to being in a wheelchair!'

I still don't think I've been through the full emotional journey, I still feel I've got a long way to go. I haven't really accepted it. I've realised the importance of having a focus and doing things rather than waiting; doing things and using that as a process to get over things. Which I suppose is something that I've been taught, the Protestant work ethic – you don't let emotions get in your way. But it's been a huge saving for me, to have had that upbringing, getting on with things, doing stuff.

So getting involved with life, having an active focus?

Yes, working, doing rather than being emotional, setting aside emotional things and getting on with doing things. The only thing I'm bad at is going too far in the doing and just totally ignoring the emotional stuff until it flies up in my face. But I think it helped me cope with things in hospital.

I went through my biggest depressing time when I was living with my aunt, in a carpeted place where I couldn't get to things and I didn't really have that much to do. There were heaps of people visiting and lots of support but I didn't have any focus. It's made such a huge difference living here and going to college, so much of my self-esteem is wrapped up with what I'm doing. Being a university student, creating and doing drawing, painting ... I've always drawn, but now the drawing has replaced the dancing.

Could you say a bit about dancing, before and after?

I realised why I danced was to make connections with people. I think that a lot of my dancing before was wrapped up with image and it's much less so now. It was always image; I'm terrible! [laughing] Dancing, I haven't done it for a while, which is bad, but it's given me a lot more movement and balance just in terms of physical stuff. If I turn on music and move for half an hour a day, which is something which I've just started doing, it makes such a huge difference to life and the way I feel; I don't feel nearly so trapped. So music and movement is still a way of getting away from stuff. I thought when I was lying in traction, 'Okay, I'm not going to be able to run away from things any more,' which is true.

But now that I'm getting all my freedoms back, I'm realising that I can again. So I think it's taught me a lot about facing things, because when I had any emotional problems I just used to go and dance, just carry on my life. But now my friendships with people have gone much deeper and stronger, just through physical necessity.

So when you'd go and dance, did that move the emotional energy that was stuck?

It would take it out; it would leave it behind and dissipate it. I'd go back to the same person and say, 'Hi, I'm back!' I'd go on my own little journey. I was quite cold to people, unlike my sister who is really so fierce about her friendships. I think that now my physical necessity is really calculated. Friendships mean so much more to me now. I suppose I was more like my mother, more about survival. My sister is always getting involved with people and helping them, she's great.

What have been the most positive things about your experience of having a disability?

The deepest, most positive thing is that until something like this happens you don't know that you can cope. And knowing that you can cope is huge; it's just such a gift of strength. But then again if I have to have an operation and I find out that I've got another complication ... you still wonder how much more you could cope with. The thought of losing my ability to speak and breathe, I didn't know whether I would be able to cope with that. That would be hard. But to know that I can cope with this much is a grounding thing, a powerful thing.

Then the whole idea of not being able to run away and having to deal with people emotionally because you are physically dependent on them; that's been really good, really enriching. The whole family is just transformed because we were really dispersed. I am closer to my family because my dependency on them is greater.

Also the faith that I've gained in people; that they will be there for you. You never know that until something like this happens. It brings me back to knowing more what my values are and to focus my life a lot more. There were so many things that I was doing, it has made me appreciate simpler things. I am less restless; you'd think it would make you more restless, it does, but in a way it doesn't.

Have there been any particular practices or techniques that you have used to facilitate your healing?

Dance has helped me a lot. Prior to my accident I was involved with a community of people. I was studying Contact Improvisation [in which] movements are motivated by two people maintaining a point of physical contact. You learn to move and to respond and you learn to open yourself up. So you go to a workshop and you sit down and talk to someone for two minutes and tell them a bit about yourself. And then suddenly your whole body is all over them, and you wouldn't know them from anyone else in the street – apart from the fact that they are the type of person who would do that sort of thing.

I was working with a dance group called Bricolage, with a dance teacher called Annetta Luce. She formed this group and we did a whole lot of performances around Sydney and really worked quite hard.

Then I started working with a woman named Janis Claxton who teaches Free and Wild at the Sydney Dance Company. She is a beautiful teacher. I studied modern dance technique with her and was working on a piece that she was choreographing at the time of my accident. I was living in a studio so I had a dance floor that was polished and Janis taught classes there. I did yoga at the Glebe Yoga School with Sue Ellen Kohler and Peter Thompson, who are amazing yoga teachers. I was studying architecture at the same time; I enrolled in all my subjects and then dis-enrolled [sic] in half of them and spent all my time dancing [laughing softly].

So that's where I was when I had my accident. And two days later my dance partner was at my bedside saying, 'Girl, we are going to choreograph a piece from Kafka and you're going to be the cockroach.'

Fantastic!

So I had that sort of support and I had Janis, and Helen Clarke Lapin, who was already working with people in wheelchairs doing Contact Improvisation. People in wheelchairs can generate movement, for instance I use my arms in a very specific way because I don't have the muscles, so there's a very different movement vocabulary there. But that's what Janis and Helen really push. I did a workshop with them. That was really confronting, to go back to the Sydney Dance Company studios and do a workshop with five of the people in the group that I used to dance with, and me in a wheelchair. It actually really refocused me and made me realise why I was dancing; what my passion for dance was. It took a lot of the ego away that I had around dance, around body. Because when I did yoga and dance it was a lot about, 'I'm going to get there and I'm going to be able to move and be really fit and healthy and strong.' A lot of determination.

Getting it right?

Yes. A lot of it was sensation-based, especially with Janis, she's really good at working with sensation energy and doing movement through finding what feels good and being really true to that, rather than copying.

So coming from the inside?

Yes, but at the same time teaching you about finding distinctions in your body. What it made me realise with dance was: it's about interacting with other people and seeing how different bodies move. It's really as simple as that. One of the most beautiful moments of the workshop was watching one able-bodied girl and one girl with paraplegia sitting on the floor moving together. [They were] dancing on the floor and it didn't matter at that point that Carol wasn't able to move her legs because they were both sitting down. And then the other girl stood up and you didn't want Carol to stand up because you just wanted to watch the way she moved differently and how she interacted with this other woman, and the difference between their movements – how beautiful Carol's movement was and how beautiful the other girl's movement was. The focus wasn't on what Carol couldn't do. It really hit home then.

> 'The deepest, most positive thing is that until something like this happens you don't know if you can cope. And knowing you can cope is such a gift of strength.'

So letting go of the comparison and just being with each individual as they express themselves.

Yes, and also just being in this position where you don't wish that that person could stand up. At that point I saw it as a positive thing, an expression of who she is. And in this context it's a beautiful thing that there's this person here who can't move her legs. It's a positive thing, completely, absolutely positive.

It's just different; it's not less.

Yes. Through dance I actually felt like I connected with other people about my experience, able-bodied people. You've got a connection with other people who are going through the same thing but it's very hard to feel like you can relate your experience to somebody else who hasn't been through it. I was halfway through the six-week workshop and I was doing this movement on the floor and Helen was trying to work with me and suddenly she said, 'Oh my God, Sara, you can't feel!' Helen knew that I could not feel but it was at this point when we were dancing together, making a connection through touch, that she connected fully with the reality of not feeling.

I was also lucky that I was comfortable with my body. I saw this fifteen-year-old girl come in to the spinal ward who was going through that awkward stage of puberty where you worry about your body and who hadn't gotten to a stage in her life where she was comfortable with her body. Then something like this happened and to have 80 different nurses looking after you, doing all the most personal care. It would have been so harrowing for her. While I was so used to running around naked and getting changed in front of people that it didn't worry me. So that was a really positive thing from dance.

There was something else I learnt from that workshop, which was that you can have as much interest in doing what we were doing as you can in doing huge things.

Like cartwheels?

Yes, like cartwheels. And that's something that Janis really works with and it can create really interesting choreography as well, something interesting to look at and something interesting to do. I also did this thing where I was put on the floor and told to move. I was given 5 square metres of mat to move on and to try and see what I could do with my body. That was incredible, that sense of freedom that I had forgotten, that I hadn't had when sitting in a chair. I haven't done that for a while actually. It's really important. It would be much healthier if my room was set up so that I rolled everywhere.

So it is more comfortable on the floor.

Yes, because you give yourself a massage while you move and your organs get massaged, which you don't get sitting in a chair. Though it's not very practical for going anywhere! Crawling on the floor ... [laughing]

I have also started having Zen shiatsu massage. I have a massage and for two days afterwards I get this shock when I look down at myself and see that I am paralysed. It's a different shock to the one I used to get when I woke up in the morning, that sickening shock of, 'I want to go back to sleep, I don't want to face it.' It's a shock that I could feel this good and be paralysed. I think shiatsu, with the whole energy balancing and the meridian stuff, has been so valuable.

But the dance and the movement has led me to connect with people physically and by doing that you realise your boundaries, realise where you can go and realise a lot about trust. I suppose my spiritual philosophy is that when you die you live on in people's memories, you live on and it's an energetic thing. You live in relation to a whole lot of people and that's spiritual, it's like this spirit that is generated by everybody and that's how we become greater than what we are individually.

> *That interconnectedness?*

I'm not good at articulating it probably because I don't think about it much. So dance becomes something spiritual in that way. You learn physically about your dependence on other people and that's emotional as well as spiritual.

> *I think you have touched on this already, but I'll ask it anyway; where do you gain your strength from?*

'I was doing this movement on the floor and Helen was trying to work with me. Suddenly she said, "Oh my God, Sara, you can't feel!"'

Knowledge of friendships, people ... when I first had my accident, I was lying there in casualty thinking, 'I don't know any of these people here but they are doing everything they can to help me.' That put a lot of faith in me. So even though there are so many problems inherent in the hospital system, still our society is set up to do that and to look after people. To be nurtured in that way is an incredible experience, it gave me lots of strength, because you have so much faith in people. So that's where I suppose a lot of people can lose strength, they lose a lot of strength because they don't have that and they don't have that experience of being nurtured, strengthened and supported.

> *So how do you understand the process of healing?*

My godmother sent me a book, *Man's Search for Meaning*. It's about this guy who went through a Nazi concentration camp, Victor Frankel. He realises that the people who've got a goal at the end can survive. I suppose the process of healing for me has been – and this is something the psychologist Geoff has helped me a lot with – finding what your values are, what you need to find meaning and then shifting your life to fulfil that so you're in line with those values. Then everything else falls away; you accept much more, I think. That whole process of acceptance is the healing process. It's really healing. I don't know whether I have actually accepted yet. I'm still really scared. I still get really scared. I think that's what the process of healing is and I still deny a lot of what I feel and run away from a lot.

> *What advice do you have for other people who have serious illness or disability?*

I think if you know what you need (it seems a very selfish way of looking at it), if you know what you value you can live that out to the very last, no matter what happens. But that's a really hard thing to know, to know what you want; it's a constant battle. I don't think you can know if you can really cope with anything unless you actually live it. I wouldn't have thought I could cope with this, and in a way it's easier to cope with the physical, your imagination is always more powerful than what the actual physical experience is.

I used to get more upset, when I first had my accident, thinking about other people thinking about what I was going through, rather than actually going through it myself, because I knew I'd be alright. I knew I'd be fine. I never lost that hope. I don't think I have really faced and taken on the hope of recovery. I think that's a very hard thing to do. I think I'd like to work on that, that takes a lot of strength. For people to truly believe that they can recover, to really lay everything on the line for that.

> *When you say recovery, what do you mean by that?*

Recovery in terms of physical recovery, to regain movement. There's a balance between, this is a soft [sic] point, being open to that possibility and still living your life. Striking that balance is really hard. There's a friend of mine who has incomplete spinal injuries and he lives with his girlfriend. She really wants him to keep pushing that edge; he goes and does physiotherapy and tries walking. But it takes four hours or more out of his day and makes him physically and emotionally exhausted. There is a point where you can't sustain that any more; you need to focus on being how you are.

I haven't had that dilemma because I don't have an incomplete injury. It's pretty cut and dried. I mean I had that initially, for six months you are told, 'Now you've got six months where it might return.' Maybe I accepted it too readily because I decided that that would be the easiest way to go, rather than fighting it. I don't think so.

There's this theory that if you fight, it's a thing of motivation; if you fight it, if you truly wished you wanted to walk, you would walk. I don't think you can possibly not have that open in you; that desire to walk and run, no matter how subconscious it is. I don't think you could ever shut yourself off from that. So long as you haven't lost your passion for life, for living. I feel really threatened when people suggest that theory. [But] there's always that wonder, if you really have accepted it too readily, and if you kick and scream more, you get more back.

> 'I used to get more upset thinking about other people thinking about what I was going through, rather than actually going through it myself, because I knew I'd be alright.'

When I asked you before about what advice you have, you said, 'Oh! I hate advice!' What did you mean by that?

Why do I hate advice? Because I've had people ask me, 'Can you give me some advice on design for people with disabilities?' I wouldn't know. I know I'm in a wheelchair but there's so many other different disabilities and different ways of coping with it and different physical needs. I suppose with advice you can take it or leave it, but the connotation of the word is that you're giving it to be taken.

Jot this down, it's authority ...

I hate the arrogance that often comes with advice. Someone signed a book for me once with; 'Be positive always and take everything that life has to offer.' I just can't cope with that.

This prescription about how to do it as opposed to lots of individuals who all do it in different ways?

Yes, the triteness, the simplistic approach, the implication that someone can generalise about an individual's experience.

Shankardev's story

From early in his life, shortness of breath, wheezing and attacks of sneezing were Shankardev's frequent companions. These continued through his adolescence and were still plaguing him when he was accepted into medical school in 1971. It was while studying in first-year medicine that Shankardev first came into contact with yoga, which he became fascinated with. He later went on to travel to India to deepen his understanding of yoga, meeting his guru Swami Satyananda in 1974. While staying at the Bihar School of Yoga in India he undertook intensive yoga practices under the guidance of his guru. Using these therapeutic applications of yoga, Shankardev was able to cure himself of his asthma and has been symptom-free since that time.

Over the last fifteen years Shankardev has been working in private practice as a doctor and yoga therapist helping people to manage chronic illnesses using yoga and Ayurveda, its sister science. I first met Shankardev in 1989 when he was working at the Wholistic [sic] Medical Centre in Surry Hills in Sydney, one of the first health care centres in Sydney whose staff included both doctors of modern medicine and various practitioners of complementary medicine. Shankardev has been actively involved in writing, researching and teaching yoga and Ayurveda over the last 25 years both in Australia and abroad. He is a much valued friend and colleague who generously shares his story for this book.

What was the nature of your condition and when did it start?

I had childhood asthma. It started when I was five or six. What I remember of it was chronic wheezing every day and allergic sneezing all the time. I felt weak and wasn't able to play and run around.

So it was incapacitating?

Yes it was, I had lots of colds, bronchitis and was always in bed. Just going into a smoky or dusty room, my eyes would start watering and I'd start sneezing and wheezing. I'd know that an attack was going to come and then would have to get through those attacks with the medications that were available at that time.

Did they have puffers then?

No, they didn't. They didn't have much; bronchitis was treated with antibiotics and I don't remember medication being very effective. I was on steroids very occasionally; everyone went on steroids. I tried to avoid that. As far as I can remember I was never hospitalised but had a very chronic condition of low energy and inability to function, and these attacks.

So it was debilitating?

Pretty debilitating, and not just debilitating but oppressive and scary, particularly the thought of having an attack. So just playing too much and laughing a lot would trigger an attack, that sense of not being able to breathe and use your lungs properly, the most horrendous feelings.

How do you think having to deal with all these symptoms affected you as a young child growing up, emotionally?

It's hard to know, it's hard to tease out cause and effect. When I look back on it all I think psychologically there was an impact, but I also think there was a two-way process; that my mind affected my body as much as my body affected my mind. As a kid you have a different view of the world. It's hard to remember how I was in those days. But certainly I was restricted in terms of my social interaction; I was shy and introverted and socially not confident to the point of even being phobic under certain circumstances. There was a real sense of inadequacy, not being able to handle school. School was hard, I think when you are sick kids pick on you a lot because you are obviously more defenceless. I think I was anxious a lot of the time.

> *So when you said that word 'phobic' before did you mean that even to think about certain situations would be too much?*

Yes, like going to school sometimes was just a horrible thought and I didn't want to face it.

> *So what would happen with your parents?*

Well, my mother was unwell so she was not very available and my father was quite distant, so there was not much interaction there. I think I was probably difficult as a child – volatile and strong-willed at times, playing up and being naughty. I think my father found that difficult. So my asthma attacks were a way of getting some emotional support. My parents would have to come forward and be more nurturing. I think that was one of the mechanisms involved in causing it to occur.

But day to day, I would just get out and play and do what I had to do; then have an attack and would come home and say 'I've had an attack.' Then they would look after me and put me to bed. It was hard on all of us. My mum was unwell, I was unwell; my dad wasn't coping either.

> *Did that situation continue when you were in high school?*

Yes, it went on through high school. I had a lot of asthma. My mother died when I was about sixteen and then, more or less, I felt I was on my own. My dad went out and led his life and I led my life; we were quite independent. Also bronchodilator inhalers became available when I was in early high school and that made a big difference.

Generally, at that time I didn't have a lot of confidence and was a little confused about life; where I was going, what I was doing socially. Recently I spoke to an old friend about that time of my life and she said I never showed it. I always had a good front but really it was very hard for me going through high school. Basically I felt like that up until university.

Throughout high school sports were difficult, interaction socially was difficult, emotionally I often felt anxious and depressed. I had a total lack of confidence about my abilities to do anything socially. Then when I was alone I would feel quite lonely, shut off and cut off from the world. Around that time I got into music, rock and roll, and started smoking marijuana in Year 10 in high school, which opened up a whole lot of avenues for me.

> *For self-expression?*

A little bit, but really it was just a kind of exploration.

> *So you finished high school and later went on to university ...*

Yes, I got through high school, somehow I made it through into medicine. I don't know how I did that.

> *So you were in medical school and you were studying health ...*

'So my asthma attacks were a way of getting emotional support. My parents would have to come forward and be more nurturing.'

Was I? In medical school ... [laughter from interviewer] not really. I think the asthma forced me to think about other options like diet, though not very seriously. Through high school I'd been interested in esoteric philosophies, Carlos Castaneda, drug culture, altered states of consciousness, that sort of thing. So health wasn't really a priority in the sense of the natural therapies approach. But when the symptoms started to come I had to start to think of what to do. I couldn't just take puffers all the time. So what actually happened, when I got into first-year medicine, was that I had a nervous breakdown. I just felt the social pressures and the drugs and my whole situation were going to kill me if I didn't do something about them.

I was quite lost. I tried to stop smoking dope and started using natural approaches to improve my health. Then I met this yoga teacher. It was around the middle of first-year university when I realised that there was something outside of the mind-altering stuff. So I started to practise yoga and started to look after my diet a bit. I started to look a bit at herbs and went to visit a few herbalists, but nothing very serious.

The yoga started to make a big impression; a strong psychological impression and I started to investigate it further. As I got more and more into yoga I realised that in order to practise it more effectively, I had to let go of the drugs at that time and change my diet and so on. So then they became more adjunctive to yoga for me.

How do you understand why you got asthma?

I think there is some hereditary component. I think I was sensitive. I'm not sure about my birth history but my family life wasn't that happy. My parents had just come out of the war in Europe and I think my mother was totally stressed out, overwhelmed, shocked and horrified. They had seen their family killed and lots of people killed. So I think that probably played a big part in it.

I think it was in my nature, in my karma, to have a weakness in the lungs. There were also stresses at that time; dietary factors such as having a Middle European type of diet, on top of a sensitive, weak constitution at birth. Then there was the emotional overlay and so on. It all plays a part.

Later on I had deep insights when I had certain experiences when I was in India; insights into how I was as a person, how I was holding myself. At the time of those insights I felt a huge shift and that's when I felt my asthma stop. I can actually remember the days though not the dates so much. There was a moment of realisation, and from that time on my body shifted and I didn't get asthma attacks. Then later on I had another realisation and my allergies stopped.

So you could see how those shifts in self-understanding affected your physical health?

Yes, it was more like a complete experience of myself. I was walking along, up the stairs once and I had this huge flash and I felt a shift take place in my body and at the same time I had this deep understanding. So it was a simultaneous thing. It was kind of strange.

A mind–body experience?

Yes, the whole thing. That is the way I'd describe it, but I can't relate that back to what was causing it as a child. I think I was born with a weak link in the chain, which was my lungs and an unhappy childhood. In a lot of ways it all came out as 'emotional constipation' I guess. That's one way of looking at it, and in Oriental medicine, the lungs, the moon and the mind are all very much connected.

> *What would you say have been the most difficult things about having asthma?*

Number one, the sense of not being able to get oxygen. You feel cut off from the life force; it's a sense of choking, you're just choking. The physical debilitation that you feel is difficult, you don't have any energy to do the things that you want to do. Every time you start to do something you get blocked by exercise-induced asthma or you can't go into certain environments, it's very limiting. It's like being an invalid. You feel totally constrained and unable to do the things you want to do.

It has a strong effect on the mind; it's very deadening, not being able to get oxygen. Your mind becomes quite dull and doesn't think clearly. Also the fear of having an asthma attack – you just don't know when it's going to happen.

'There was a moment of realisation, and from that time on I didn't get asthma attacks. Later on I had another realisation and my allergies stopped.'

When bronchodilators came in, that made a big difference to my wellbeing and lifestyle, a huge difference. I remember that each week I knew that I was going to have a couple of attacks at least and they could come any time; and when they did come it affected your quality of life. It was very embarrassing just being with people, you had to have inhalers with you and you've got to go and puff; they see that you're weak and that triggers the feelings of social inadequacy.

> *So having bronchodilators gave you a greater sense of being in control?*

Yes, but they didn't always work and I also had a lot of allergies, which were a big component of it as well; dust, animals, smoke, pollens, foods. I had testing when I was a kid and I got injections to try and desensitise me but they didn't work at all, in my opinion. So it wasn't just the asthma, it was the allergies as well, they were a big part of my experience of illness.

What would you say have been the most positive things about having had asthma?

Looking back now? I think the positive part of it was learning to get out of it. Learning yoga, learning about life and accepting life as it is and then finding my strength to climb out. There is nothing positive about having asthma in itself. You definitely get compassion for people; they are suffering and you are suffering yourself, so as I got older and as I was studying medicine, you definitely have a deeper sense of understanding of what other people are going through. So maybe there is more empathy that comes out of it. But the true positive thing for me was the capacity to find a way to manage it more effectively and to cure it, to finish it off.

So how did that process come about?

Through yoga, mainly. I went to India and underwent rigorous yogic training, including a lot of saltwater cleansing, in an ashram in Bihar in India. By 1974–75 I was doing three hours of meditation each morning including an hour and a half of *pranayama* [yogic breathing], plus I was doing intensive body cleansing, saltwater cleansing using *lagoo, kunjal* and *neti*.

Could you say a little more about those practices?

Yes, sure. But just to backtrack a little before I talk about that. What happened was that I started studying yoga in 1971 at university. Then some swamis came out from the Bihar School of Yoga around '73 and I started to practise their style of yoga, which included a lot more *pranayama*, a lot more meditation, introduction to spiritual philosophy and the concept of guru. That in itself was probably one of the most profound catalysts. To feel the connection to a guru and to recognise the possibility of that was much more important than the actual *asanas* [postures] and the *pranayama* and the saltwater cleansing.

So you felt a strong connection with a teacher …

A teacher with a lineage, a tradition and with the whole Indian approach to yoga and the yogic philosophies that come out with yoga. I felt very at home with them. I had a lot of experiences of that, even before I was at university. In 1969 when I was seventeen I went out to a nightclub and met a girl there who had come back from India, who had shaved her head and had a ring in her nose. I had no idea what that was all about but felt some connection and she was fascinating. So I actually used that as a way to introduce myself, like: 'Where did you get the ring? What's going on? Why did you shave your the head?' She said: 'Oh, I've just come back from India and I'm working here to get enough money to go back.' So I said: 'I'm very interested in that, do you want to talk about it?' I went back to her place and she showed me Swami Vivekananda's book on Raj yoga and that was the first yoga book I got my hands on.

So the philosophy was actually my introduction to yoga and then I started to develop an interest through esoteric stuff. I was interested in black magic, I read a bit of Alistair Crowley. But drugs were a consistent part of my life up until university. Then I met this yoga teacher at the university, he had a real serenity and inner glow; and just the sense of him being so self-contained, that was impressive.

> 'I met this yoga teacher at the university; he had a real serenity and inner glow. Just the sense of him being so self-contained was impressive.'

So all of that led up to my connection with Swami Satyananda. I'd been doing a lot of practice, especially *asana* and *pranayama*, prior to the connection to Swamiji. Then I went to India in 1974, started to practise Kriya yoga, and went through a profound detoxification process. The Kriya practices were very intense.

These are breathing practices?

It's a series of techniques using breath and visualisation and the hatha yoga *bandhas* [techniques that involve stopping the flow of energy in a localised part of the body] and *mudras* [hand gestures used in yoga postures and meditation] to charge the body. I actually wasn't fully prepared for this, I just wanted to jump in the deep end but I had a really huge detox.

When you say you had a huge detox, what do you mean?

Well, I got quite ill. I had a whole lot of symptoms. I had a lot of asthma, fevers, diarrhoea, boils, a lot of symptoms of overheating from the practices. But I stayed there for three months the first time and in that three-month period I learnt the first ten *kriyas* [techniques used in yoga that involve modifying one's breath and visualising certain images]. There are twenty *kriyas* in all. I learnt the first ten and practised them diligently for a year when I got back. I recovered from those illnesses. I was basically resilient underneath the asthma.

I then went back to India in 1975 for six months. I had a big term break from university and in that time I learnt the rest of the *kriyas*. I had a huge reaction then and again became very sick. I was lying in bed unable to move, basically my bronchitis was very bad and my asthma was very bad. I just remember feeling that yoga was hopeless. I was thinking, 'This is just not working. I'll go back to Australia and just concentrate on orthodox medicine.'

Then I had this huge out-of-body experience while lying in bed. I just saw myself ... It was quite a profound experience, very hard to talk about but a realisation of something at a deep level, and I got better and that was the last of my asthma. That was it; that was the last major attack I had.

So Kriya yoga had been the primary process and I had been diligent, terribly disciplined, rigidly disciplined, obsessive. Along with that, I'd been doing hatha yoga cleansing techniques, saltwater cleansing, which means drinking six glasses of water, washing the bowel. I'd use *kunjal* every time I had an attack, and I had a lot of attacks while I was practising Kriya yoga. I had been doing the Kriya yoga up until 1976, when I had my last attack. The *kunjal* I'd used to clean the body.

So the kunjal *involves?*

Saltwater cleansing, drinking six glasses of salty water and then putting the fingers into the throat and gagging and bringing up all the water out of the stomach. Followed by *neti;* cleansing the nasal passages. I used that when I was okay to maintain my health but also whenever I had an acute attack of asthma, to try and break the attack rather than using any medication. I'd use the *kunjal* and hot black coffee, those kind of things and a lot of natural therapies by that time.

You mean you drank black coffee?

Yes, because it's a bronchodilator. So the yoga was primary but I'd also been using a lot of herbs, a lot of diet. I'd experimented with all sorts of diet – mucus-less diet, raw foods, macrobiotics – I'd done all of that up until that period of doing yoga, up until 1976 when I was lying in bed and had that attack, which was the last. That was a major breakthrough in which I had a vision of what yoga potentially could do but also how much was required to get to that depth. I had been living in an ashram for six months; I'd been practising three hours of yoga daily. I was living a very rigorous lifestyle and connected up with a teacher who could guide me through a lot of the emotional blockages. All of that was required, I believe, to make that deep shift.

> So living with somebody who was wise and a strong role model?

Yes, absolutely; plus someone who understood the process, who understood what was required to heal, who had that knowledge of healing the mind–body through yoga. So a lot of *asana*, a lot of *pranayama*, then Kriya yoga and then herbs and diets. I'd seen lots of naturopaths and I was reading and studying a lot, whatever I could get my hands on.

> So through this whole process of healing that took place over quite a few years, where would you say you got your strength from?

'I'm talking about deep insight into self; self-awareness and then the capacity to manipulate yourself in a way that takes you towards greater healing, health and wholeness.'

I'm just very determined as a person, I believe; obsessive. I have this kind of tenacious character. So when I put my mind to something I will do anything. For personal goals such as to get through medicine, it requires a certain tenacity, discipline and to some degree I've had that in some ways I guess. Inspiration from Swamiji, my teacher, was a big part of that. There were times when I wanted to quit; I think he probably inspired me to keep going.

> What have you learnt through the experience of having asthma?

So much, it's a big question. Self-healing, along with the study of medicine, has taken up most of my life. What happened to me when I had that experience in India, in Christmas of 1975 – that breakthrough into a deep understanding of myself – that's part of my yoga. The healing I see as secondary to the yoga. The insight, the yoga, is the primary thing; the healing is secondary.

So when you are talking about yoga ...

I'm talking about deep insight into self; self-awareness, self-knowledge and then the capacity to manipulate oneself in a way which takes one towards greater healing and towards greater health and wholeness.

Then there were stages after that, when I had another experience, when I went back to India the year after. I was staying in the ashram and while walking up these stairs I just had an allergic reaction. I wasn't wheezing but I started sneezing, my eyes were watering again, I'd just been in a dusty environment, I felt weakened. Then I had another insight, though not as strong as the previous experience. So in the process of the illness, in the process of suffering, a lot of insights can come about.

That was the last time I had a severe allergic reaction, in the nature of a runny nose, watering eyes, sneezing and all that. When I came back, I actually had myself tested [at a leading teaching hospital], not that year, but later on. I had histamine challenges, and all my tests were normal.

So yoga was primary, the healing was secondary. The health of the body, the asthma, was secondary to becoming self-aware and the recognition of that possibility in me. Also at a personal level, a recognition that it's a weak link and that I've always got to look after my health; that I've got a sensitive nature and that I've got to maintain it and find ways to do that. I'm quite driven in a lot of ways – to achieve things and to be successful – and that puts a lot of wear and tear on my body. So I've got to do a lot of yoga as a way of balancing out.

So I've learnt to balance my life to stay healthy, to get healthier as I get on, to recognise the things that work for me and that therefore I can share with others. The Ayurveda, herbalism, bodywork, massage, counselling, psychotherapy, acupuncture, all those other modalities, which I've personally tested on myself. Modalities that I have an experience of and that I use for myself to maintain my health.

But primarily, more and more yoga comes back. Its capacity to generate vitality, mental peace and tranquillity. Insight, too, to learn to accept myself, to be myself and to use that just to be who I am, to live this life and to live it out. To live out the drama of it, the scenario, the scenes, whatever arises, and then to share whatever I've got with others. Again I think there has been a strong empathy for others, through my mother's death when I was a child and then my own illness. There has been a focus on health and healing, psychological as well as physical healing, over the years – that's been a big focus. Out of that I've developed a capacity to guide others and to help them to become stronger if they choose to follow a path similar to the one I have experienced.

> So in your work as a doctor and yoga therapist you are actively drawing from that reservoir of experience in helping other people with chronic illnesses?

Absolutely, and also a big part of it is my relationship with my guru, with Swamiji. How his training and his influence have been fundamental in giving me guidelines, structures and methods to express that knowledge in a way that is relatively effective. Knowledge of healing, knowledge of yoga, knowledge of healing arts and how to combine those things in a way that's simple but effective.

'Healing is mind, body and consciousness, of which consciousness is the most important. The more one rests in consciousness, the less it matters whether your body is healthy or not.'

> This is something that you have touched on but I'd like to ask you anyway; how do you understand the process of healing, given your experiences?

Well, I understand healing now in a multidimensional way. I think that I have the capacity to heal myself, but I don't think everybody does. I think there are limits, and I also have limits of things that I also can't change. Even though I've stopped my asthma, there are still limits on my vitality.

As I understand healing now, there is self-healing and finding methods to generate your own vitality and mental wellbeing, knowledge and insight. The synthesising of information to [gain] a progressively more enlightened understanding of life and self and the relationships.

Also the capacity to bring external modalities to bear, that's part of it.

Healing is mind, body and consciousness, of which consciousness is probably the most important. Ultimately, the more one rests in consciousness the less it matters so much whether your body is healthy or unhealthy. The second most important is mental stability and the third most important is physical health.

So healing is the capacity to address the three levels, it is the capacity to pinpoint the issues that are relevant to the particular condition that you are looking at. It's also the capacity to see that within the whole, how that fits into the whole structure of one's self, one's family, society, self-expression, allowing life back in, in terms of emotional relationship and nourishment at all levels. It is such a big question.

At a more pragmatic level, what advice do you have for other people who are facing serious illness?

Practise yoga! [smiling] Find out what's appropriate for you. Investigate as many methods and methodologies as you can in order to find your own way. Get information, get educated, apply things, use the illness as a springboard into higher awareness, understanding of life. Try to see that illness has a validity – it's a valid part of existence; it's an essential part of existence – and work towards greater health at all levels, primarily spiritual ... health of consciousness.

It's a very complex issue; we are talking within the social context we live in, a sick society in my opinion. A society that has lost its values, that has become sensory driven; a society that is material and consuming, polluting, more and more selfish. So health has to be seen in the broader context, as much as in the individual. I think that a lot of the ill health we experience is as a result of the world that we have created and how we live. So it just goes on ...

To find meaning, to use your illness to find meaning and whatever works for you as an individual, then that's the way through it for you. I think yoga has its application to all forms of chronic illness: whether it's in learning to relax more deeply; whether it's learning to observe the mind through meditation, which is part of yoga; whether it's just finding ways to breathe a little bit more efficiently, to circulate blood, calm the nerves, relax muscle and send *prana* through the body, to circulate *prana*.

It can be very simple, it can be used anywhere; it can be used in a hospital bed, in an intensive care ward, anywhere.

So if I had a personal message it would be to be open-minded to yoga and to see beyond the limitations of its present definition in our society, which is as a very robust form of stretching and *asana* – to see it as a model for self-exploration and self-awareness.

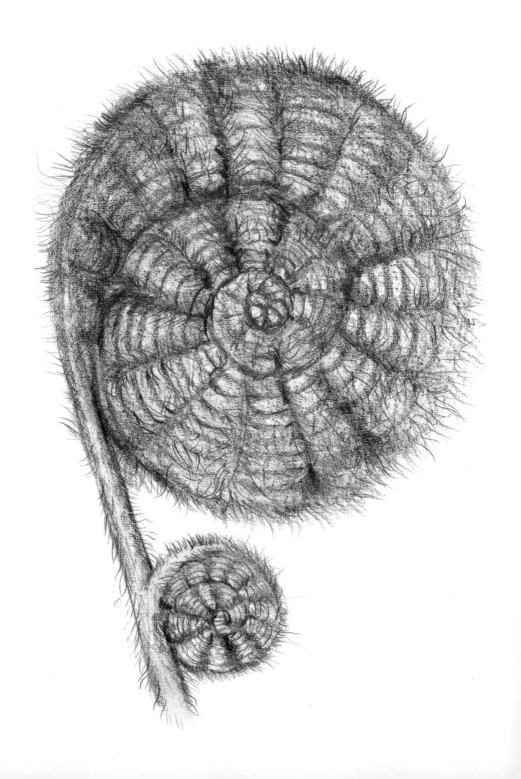

What we can learn

PART II

The crosier (unfurled frond) of an Australian tree fern, symbolising the unfolding nature of the process of healing and the need for ongoing growth even in maturity

Getting proactive

'You have to fall in love with your disease to a degree, so that it doesn't become something that you leave in the too-hard basket.'
NICKI YOUDALE

A common question asked of me by people not familiar with complementary medicine is: 'Does it work?' My answer, which is not usually what they are expecting, is: 'It depends on the individual.' From my experience in clinical practice I can definitely say that those individuals who get actively involved in creative ways in their own recovery do get very positive results. In this chapter I want to address this principle of self-responsibility, which is so powerfully evident in the stories of the eight people interviewed in this book.

Faced with the diagnosis of a serious illness, it is quite natural for most of us to go into some kind of shock. Our most cherished images of ourselves and our future lives are immediately confronted, the whole situation can seem quite unreal initially. At this juncture we will often feel out of control and emotionally vulnerable. When working as a resident doctor in an acute coronary care unit I well remember seeing the lost look on the faces of middle-aged men admitted with heart attacks. Men used to being powerful in the outside world in their capacities as managing directors or lawyers were now in fear for their lives, hooked up to various beeping monitors, restricted to bed and dependent on nurses to bring bedpans, meals and even the telephone.

The loss of health, like any kind of loss in our lives, is accompanied by a complex set of emotional reactions that differ enormously from person to person and in the same person over time. The writings of Dr Elisabeth Kübler-Ross [a Swiss-born psychiatrist, now living in the US, whose pioneering work in the field of death and the process of dying shaped modern medical understanding] in differentiating the stages in the process of grieving loss has certainly informed my understanding of how people react to the diagnosis of serious illness. Based on her experience of working with people with major loss in their lives, she distinguishes the stages of shock, denial, anger, bargaining, depression and acceptance that individuals experience after loss. These reactions do not necessarily follow a linear sequence and people can sometimes get stuck at one particular stage for long periods of time.

'Grieving needs to be an active process whereby we give ourselves time to allow it to unfold in its own way'

I mention these stages to give some kind of context to what the individuals interviewed in this book have been able to achieve. Their capacity to move through the enormous amount of loss involved in being seriously ill is no less than extraordinary. I say extraordinary, as it is my experience that contemporary Western society does not know how to grieve well. Too often there is considerable pressure to get back to work and 'get on with life' in ways that do not allow people to acknowledge their pain and the feelings they are left with after an important loss. In this environment heartfelt issues will often tend to go underground, playing themselves out in people's lives in ways that can undermine their health and wellbeing. Grieving needs to be an active process whereby we give ourselves time to allow the process to unfold in its own individual way. This is where the rituals of ancient cultures carry a lot of wisdom and facilitate a more healthy approach to the ubiquitous human experience of loss.

What do we mean by self-responsibility?

In order to answer this question we need look no further than the story of Nicki Youdale and how she has been able to maintain her health and wellbeing despite having a severe congenital heart disease that was expected to claim her life before her teenage years. After seeing how the recipients of heart-lung transplants waiting to see their doctors looked, Nicki was determined to find another way. So began an arduous but ultimately rewarding journey, which by her own reckoning was motivated more by a fear of the heart-lung transplant operation than of dying. It was this fear, coupled with her implicit understanding that no-one else was going to heal her other than herself, that drove her recovery. Importantly, Nicki's determination to stay with her chosen path is striking. She talks of how, initially, none of the natural therapeutic approaches seemed to be helping her and I imagine it would have been very tempting to chuck the whole thing in and go back to her heart specialists. However, she continued to stay open to the possibility of another way and later met a doctor who started her on a strict dietary, vitamin and herbal therapeutic program to which she attributes her good health for the next five years.

Nicki's approach illustrates an attitude to health and wellbeing that is fundamentally self-responsible. She is basically respectful of her physicians, recognising their expertise and experience, but clearly realises that her long-term survival on the planet is also in her own hands. Modern Western medicine has undoubtedly served her well during her life and she has a warm relationship with her heart specialist, but ultimately she knows that she too is an important decision maker in how to best manage her health. This basic position underlies the stories of all the individuals I interviewed and is evident in the patients in my clinical practice who do well.

Peter de Reuter also makes this point, advocating the importance of educating yourself and indeed becoming your own authority when it comes to managing your health. He warns of the dangers of depending on only one medical system and promotes staying open to other sources of knowledge about healing. This approach is echoed by Janelle Meisner, who advises people faced with serious illness to get 'lots of different opinions from all different types of cultural expressions of illness'. In her own case Traditional Chinese Medicine's eloquent descriptions of her condition were much more helpful and holistic in their appraisal of her illness. Rather than having her illness attributed to dysfunction in a specific organ, it emphasised her relationship to the wider world and the concept of building harmony in her life. Its approach was far more accessible and empowering; not focusing on what is wrong but on how to create balance and harmony.

In order for the individuals interviewed for this book to search beyond the realms of mainstream Western medicine, a fundamental shift had to take place in their thinking. This involved them taking control in terms of how best to create the necessary conditions for healing to take place. This does not mean disregarding the advice and treatment strategies offered by their doctors; indeed it is apparent that many of those interviewed hold their doctors and their advice in high esteem. Rather, they acknowledge that no one system holds all the answers and that it is in their own best interests to look further afield. The locus of control rests with them rather than their physicians, helping them to feel empowered and in control of their lives.

What does 'getting proactive' mean in practical terms?

When we look at the experience of the eight people interviewed we get a more concrete sense of what is meant by 'getting proactive'. All eight have moved beyond the state of denial, that tendency in all of us to think that if I just keep doing what I'm doing everything will work out alright – the proverbial 'She'll be right, mate!' attitude, as Nicki Youdale described it. Nicki sheds further light on this attitude that can so often limit the possibility of a more engaged and active approach to one's own healing when she talks about getting to a place where one feels more at ease with one's mortality. Once one can reach that place inside oneself then the next step of asking the question 'Okay, now what can I do?' becomes possible.

Another place where people can get stuck along the road to recovery is alluded to by Peter de Reuter when he says of illness: '[It's] an opportunity or a curse. You can use your condition to either grow or to become totally self-absorbed and indulgent.' For people who are unable to move beyond the anger stage of the loss of their health, it is often easy to feel a victim of life. As Peter later points out, you can then use your illness to manipulate people around you, in ways that are ultimately self-destructive and debilitating to your own life force.

Nicki Youdale advocates asking plenty of questions at the time of the consultation with your health care practitioner. Many of my patients arrive with a set of questions written down and obviously have a set of goals for what they want to get out of their consultation. Other patients come to see me after seeking help from a variety of other health care professionals and have actively been shopping around for a practitioner who shares their personal style and philosophy for a considerable period of time. Both these groups of patients have developed skill in getting the most out of the medical system. Like Nicki, their approach is assertive while still being respectful of their physician.

It is easy for people to feel intimidated by doctors and their busy schedules, but ultimately they are being paid, either directly or indirectly, by you to help you get better. In this context it is only appropriate that you fully understand what is being said to you and are made aware of implications of the treatments that are being prescribed and the different therapeutic options available. Having a close friend or relative present at the consultation can be very helpful in making sure your prepared questions are asked and in remembering what was said by the doctor or complementary medical practitioner. Asking permission from the practitioner to tape record the consultation can also be a useful strategy when you are on your own.

For all of those interviewed it has also meant seeking help from various forms of complementary medical practitioners. Janelle, Rebecca and Shankardev have received enormous help from approaches to healing from non-Western cultures, drawing heavily from Traditional Chinese Medicine, Ayurveda and yoga. Anna Rivers benefited greatly from Vipassana meditation, a Burmese Buddhist meditation practice. For some people consulting a complementary medical practitioner, often from a medical tradition about which they know very little, is a huge step. My own first visit to see an acupuncturist, only a few years after graduating from medical school, was probably only made possible by the fact that she was the mother of a close friend of mine. My friend's relaxed explanations of what happens in a consultation helped to overcome my fear that a collapsed lung from an inadvertently placed needle was only a hair's breadth away! Happily, acupuncture has been a faithful friend to me ever since that time, helping me through many difficult moments when my health was suffering and Western medicine had little to offer me.

From his experience of struggling to keep his immune system strong against the HIV virus, Peter de Reuter advocates searching for information about illness beyond the usual mainstream sources. The ability of health care consumers to access information through the Internet on the latest developments in the treatment of all manner of medical conditions obviously greatly facilitates this process in the twenty-first century. Another practical way of being proactive which has been useful for some of the individuals interviewed is attending illness support groups. Janelle Meisner, in particular, alludes to how useful it was for her in dealing with chronic fatigue syndrome to realise that: 'I can be helped, too, and it is okay. These people are just normal people like me and they have been helped.' Making the effort to go to these meeting places, often run at night in a distant suburb or a twenty-minute drive into town, or to spend several hours on the Internet exploring a myriad of websites, is part of what it means to be proactive.

In the cases of Rebecca Hutchinson, Sara Chesterman and Janelle Meisner, one aspect of being proactive was a willingness to commit themselves, in terms of time and money, to lengthy periods of weekly psychotherapy. They all describe how much strength they drew from the therapists they worked with at different stages in their recoveries.

Psychological underpinnings

Having looked at some of the practical expressions of how the individuals interviewed for this book have taken responsibility for their health, I would now like to turn our attention to some of the psychological qualities that underpin their actions. The first quality I want to give some attention to could best be described as an openness to different ways or treatments that may enhance healing. This quality is especially evident in the way all eight people interviewed have been actively listening for possible approaches to facilitate their own wellbeing.

Following her intuition, Anna Rivers decided to learn how to meditate. At the time she was learning t'ai chi, and the word 'meditating' came up. She decided that if meditation was good enough for the ancient sages, it might be good for her, too. As she says, 'So that little seed was planted that this meditating thing was a good thing.' From that listening for a possibility as to how best to repair the rent in the fabric of her mind came her interest in Vipassana meditation, which she continues to this day and which she feels has been the foundation of her healing.

Nicki Youdale's willingness to stay open to possible ways to improve her lung function led her to try the Buteyko breathing technique, which has now become one of the pillars of her daily health routine. Janelle Meisner ventured into somatic psychotherapy, which brought greater levels of awareness of her own body. This awareness helped her to better understand why she got sick and how she could improve her health.

The second quality I would like to examine, which seems to go hand in hand with being proactive, involves the capacity to stay true to the process of self-healing despite its difficulties. Shankardev Saraswati's story illustrates this point well. He vividly describes the major turning point in his asthmatic condition that came while lying ill in bed with serious asthma and bronchitis in an ashram in India. Shankardev recalls feeling that yoga, which had become an enormous support to his health both mentally and physically, was hopeless and thinking that he should pack his bags and return to Australia. It was at this time that he had an out-of-body experience, which heralded a profound level of healing of the 'bodymind' [a term that acknowledges the innate connection between the mind and body] and the end of his asthma. But this 'healing crisis' came after years of training in yoga postures, breathing exercises and meditation and cleansing practices during which he had several aggravations of his asthma and other untoward symptoms. Rather than throw in the towel at these times, Shankardev persisted with these self-healing practices in the face of initial setbacks and was duly rewarded for his tenacity. The idea that a crisis point can also be an opportunity for healing at the deepest levels is supported by naturopathic theory and practice and is echoed by several of the individuals interviewed.

In keeping with Shankardev's powerful commitment to his own healing, the necessity of doing whatever it takes to facilitate healing is also made clear by Nicki Youdale, who says: 'If you really want to have the opportunity to experience some lovely things in your life, you're not going to do it unless you do the hard work first, and the hard work is bloody hard.' This will necessarily involve moving out of our comfort zones, facing our fears and opening ourselves to new experiences.

Obviously this will mean different things to different people. For some it may be seeing a psychotherapist for the first time in their lives, for others it may be being with the loneliness of staying at home on a Saturday night when all your friends are out drinking. Sara Chesterman recounts how confronting it was for her to go back to the Sydney Dance Company studios to do '... a workshop with five of the people in the group that I used to dance with, and me in a wheelchair.' As it transpired, this act of raw courage was a catalyst in, as she says, making her realise why she really loved dancing. It also enabled her to move into a whole new relationship with dance, despite her quadriplegia.

The link between being proactive and having better health

We have looked at the various ways in which the individuals interviewed for this book have been actively involved in promoting their own healing. But how is this able to affect something as tangible as their physical health? Here my understanding has been influenced by two schools of thought, one ancient and one modern. Both Ayurveda and the emerging field in Western medicine called psychoneuroimmunology have some powerful insights into how the mind affects bodily functioning.

Ayurveda

In the case of Ayurveda, one of the central principles governing how it understands health and disease is called *agni*. *Agni* is a Sanskrit word that means 'fire'; it is the biological fire responsible for the metabolic functioning of the human body. It refers to the sacred fire within all of us that is responsible for transformation; the transformation that takes place when we ingest an apple and a few hours later it becomes part of our flesh and bones. This principle of *agni* is so important that it has been worshipped in India over thousands of years and there are still many Indians today who practise *agnihotra* or fire worship on a daily basis.

In the context of the human being, *agni* expresses itself on two levels:

the physical and the mental. On the physical level it refers to the physical process of digestion; the process that enables us to draw sustenance from the food we consume. On the mental level it refers to our power of discernment, our capacity to draw nourishment from the everyday experiences of our lives. The concept of *agni* explains why a difficult experience, such as having a serious illness, can become for some people a pathway for a deeper understanding of life and for others an experience that leaves them feeling hard done by and ripped off. From the perspective of Ayurveda, the physical and mental aspects of our *agni*, our 'digestive' capacity, mirror each other with remarkable accuracy.

The physical aspect of *agni* exists in the digestive tract, the liver and in the tissues of our bodies. Ayurveda describes the functioning of the *agni* using simple and elegant metaphors derived from nature, which we can use to illumine our understanding of the functioning of our bodyminds. In this metaphor the stomach and small intestines are seen as a pot for the food we eat, food is then cooked by the action of hydrochloric acid and various enzymes that break down food as well as bile secreted by the liver. If our *agni* is balanced, we will be well able to break down, absorb and assimilate the food we eat. If it is out of balance in some way, our food will not be properly cooked and will enter into our bodies in an undigested form. This has important ramifications for our health, as this improperly digested food is said to create toxins in the body, known as *ama*. *Ama* is said to be the root of all disease and affects the proper functioning of our immune system.

The end product of the process of digestion is the nutrient fluid that gets absorbed into our bodies; we can liken this fluid to a soup that bathes all the cells of our body. Ayurveda holds that the quality of this soup will determine the state of the nourishment of our tissues in general. If we have eaten a wholesome meal, cooked with love, in relaxed surroundings and with people whose company we enjoy we will reap the benefits. Obviously this is very different to rushing down takeaway food while on the run and with our mind elsewhere. In simple terms, the nutrition of our bodies can only be as good as the quality of the nutrient soup – what we call the plasma in modern-day parlance – that bathes the tissues in our bodies. In this way the *agni* of the digestive tract is directly related to the *agni* at the level of our tissues, including our immune system. *Agni* also exists in the liver as the enzymes responsible for neutralising cancer-producing chemicals called carcinogens, and is responsible for the production of antibodies that are released into the bloodstream to destroy unwanted bacteria and viruses.

At the mental level *agni* refers to our intelligence, understanding and perception. It determines our capacity to make sense of the different experiences that come our way in life. Experiences that we are able to digest allow us to grow and become more whole as human beings. Experiences that we are not able to digest can lead to the build-up of mental toxins. These toxins may manifest as a souring in our attitude towards life and the build-up of resentment and bitterness towards other people. This tends to depress our *agni* further, leading to more accumulation of mental and emotional residues and distortion of our perception of events in life.

'Life comes along in all its various shapes and forms. What is our capacity to digest these experiences?'

When we are chronically angry or depressed, naturally our *agni* gets disturbed; if the imbalance goes on for long enough it may manifest later as some form of chronic disease. Here again we come back to the concept of digestion in the broadest sense of the word. Life comes along in all its various shapes and forms. What is our capacity to digest these experiences? We have all experienced situations in our lives that were difficult to digest, perhaps the death of a close friend or family member or the breakup of a relationship that meant a lot to us. When these difficult experiences happen to us, are we able to draw nourishment from them or do they engender bitterness or leave us with a sour taste in our mouths? Here *agni* refers to the power of discernment: what is our capacity to deal with all the vagaries of life that come our way? How able are we to draw nourishment from seemingly difficult experiences? Do we collapse into depression when we lose our job or do we see it as an opportunity to create a more satisfying livelihood for ourselves?

Clearly the eight individuals interviewed, despite the obvious hardships involved, have used their illnesses as vehicles for growth and self-understanding. They have taken a proactive stance in relation to their illnesses; by participating actively in their own healing they derive the benefits of feeling more empowered in the domain of their personal health. Rather than taking a passive approach to their recovery, at the whim of external forces beyond their control, they have taken responsibility for their own healing. This has entailed enlisting help from various quarters but essentially putting themselves in the driver's seat. From an Ayurvedic perspective, these journeys of healing have helped to balance their *agnis*, at both the physical and mental levels. When one's *agni* is more balanced, the immune system is better able to do what it is designed to do. Thus we can see how this ancient tradition of healing neatly brings together the quality of our mental processes and the quality of our physical health. In this way, being proactive and having better physical health are inherently related.

Psychoneuroimmunology

In the last 30 years modern medical science has increasingly come to the same conclusion, though the methodology has been very different. Psychoneuroimmunology, an emerging field of study and clinical practice in Western medicine, is beginning to make its mark. It is directly concerned with how the mind influences the nervous and endocrine systems, which in turn influences the immune system. There is now a considerable body of scientific evidence documenting the connections between the mind and the body. The body's 'stress hormone', cortisol, has long been known to directly affect immune system functioning. Recent research has shown that there are receptor sites for chemical messengers produced by the brain (called neuropeptides) on the surface of our white blood cells – the same cells that are responsible for fighting off infections and destroying aberrant cancer cells. It has also been found that our white blood cells, once activated, can produce substances (called interleukins and interferons) that can be perceived by our brain. In this way our immune system cells can 'talk' to our nervous system and some researchers are referring to the immune system as a part of the brain 'floating in the body'. Modern scientific research is also pointing to the fundamental links between the body and the mind, and implicit in this view is that the quality of our thoughts directly affects the quality of our immune system functioning. For readers who are interested to know more on this subject I include a list of suggested readings in mind–body medicine in the 'Further reading' section of this book. Suffice to say, the correlations between the latest advances in medical research, the wisdom of the ancient Indian yogis and those individuals interviewed in this book are striking.

* * * * * *

I would like to conclude by drawing our attention to the quote from Nicki Youdale that I chose to preface this chapter: 'You have to fall in love with your illness to a degree, so that it doesn't become something that you leave in the too-hard basket.' I find her words describing the process whereby one moves into a fundamentally different relationship with one's illness to be particularly apt. When we fall in love with someone, our thinking is profoundly affected. Thoughts about the last time we were together, what they said and the things we would like to share with them are all circulating in our minds incessantly. In short, we bring an enormous level of attention to bear on that person. My sense of what Nicki is saying here is that we need to intensely focus on our illness in order to bring about change. This does not mean wallowing in our misfortune in a self-obsessed way but rather thinking and questioning about how best to facilitate our recovery. Only then can we really equip ourselves for the journey ahead.

Living with serious illness

'It was like everything I thought I was, was being unravelled.'
REBECCA HUTCHINSON

In this chapter I would like to explore the many dimensions of what it's like to live with a serious illness. As the quote from Rebecca Hutchinson highlights, having a serious illness can be a profound threat to our innate sense of ourselves and who we are in the world. For someone who is used to being able to travel through life with robust good health, having a serious illness can seem like a fall from grace as one is confronted with the multiple losses inherent in being seriously ill. These losses are well described in the stories in Part I.

As many people's self-identity is inextricably tied up with their livelihood, loss of health and the impact it has on our ability to continue in our normal work can be devastating. For some of those interviewed, continuing in their usual job was simply impossible. In the case of Rebecca, as the symptoms of chronic fatigue syndrome became worse she was unable to sustain the intensity of her work as a book editor in a busy publishing company. She recounts how stopping work was a huge blow to her because so much of her self-esteem was tied up in her chosen career. This point is mirrored in the experience of Janelle Meisner when she says: 'What was very difficult was that I had got lots of kudos in my life from being busy, successful and organising things and now I was not able to do really anything at all.'

Rebecca also describes how confronting it was for her to go on social security benefits; in her world at that time this was a course of action for people who had failed in some way, reinforcing her sense of herself as a failure for getting sick. She said she felt that only weak people get sick. Being dependent and incapacitated is so often counter to our images of what it means to be strong. Getting sick can then become perfect fuel for the voice of our internal critic and all the 'if only' statements. 'If only I'd exercised more. If only I'd been more careful with my diet. If only I'd listened to my intuition. If only I'd got out of that relationship!' And so we can condemn ourselves to months or years of self-torment and anguish.

> 'Being dependent, incapacitated and vulnerable is so often counter to our images of what it means to be strong'

This inherent tendency to give ourselves a hard time for getting sick has unfortunately been reinforced by some New Age thinking, which sees us as creating our illnesses through our thinking. As Anna Rivers points out in her interview, this is an all too simplistic equation that isn't quite true. The corollary of this equation is that if we are lying dying from our illness then in some way we have failed. What is so tragic here is that such an attitude can profoundly disrupt the acceptance of the process of dying, an essentially natural process.

The destructive effect of this glib approach to understanding the causes of illness is also echoed in the experience of Rebecca Hutchinson. In the midst of her battle to overcome chronic fatigue syndrome she was confronted with comments from people who saw her problem as some kind of spiritual block. Given her vulnerability and confusion at the time it was easy for her to judge herself harshly, wondering if really she had some deep problem in her psyche and that she didn't really want to get better.

Often this line of thought only serves to kindle more self-loathing and judgement. Rebecca recalls her turmoil when people suggested that her illness was a spiritual block. The fact that she couldn't sit and meditate became a spiritual problem, which indicated that she wasn't very far on the path. Her judgements about herself at the time: 'Am I creating this illness? Do I not want to get better enough?' only added to her suffering.

Friends, family and intimate relationships

Often other people's judgements make matters worse for the person who is sick and contribute to our sense of shame around developing an illness. Anna Rivers recalls how difficult it was for her to speak about her illness because of the stigma of mental illness in our society and because of comments she received at times from friends who were unable to acknowledge her struggle. At a later point in her healing she talks of how important it was for her to acknowledge her mental breakdown, to be able to say, 'Look, I'm just not an ordinary person, I've had this thing happen. But it's alright. It's okay.' It was not until six years after her illness that Anna was able to begin to talk about what was for her a defining moment in her life.

In this context, we can see how serious illness can lead to wanting to withdraw from our normal social life and from people in general. Indeed this has been the experience of a number of the people interviewed, serious illness bringing the loss of connection to friends and family. Peter de Reuter, after being given his diagnosis of being HIV positive over the telephone, had enormous difficulty in sharing his news with friends. Many of them were so disturbed by the significance of his diagnosis that they needed to be counselled and supported themselves. Not surprisingly, with this kind of reception Peter learnt to stop sharing his truth with others and to find solace in other ways.

Janelle Meisner also describes how unsupportive some of her friends and family were during her illness and how difficult it was for them to accept that she was not like she used to be. She mentions that at times they became irritated with her; she was told to pull up her sleeves and to get on with life. Being surrounded with these types of attitudes where one feels misunderstood can, as Janelle goes on to say, make relationships difficult. The natural tendency is then to withdraw from those people and to feel isolated.

Rebecca also talks of how difficult relationships can become and being in the double bind of 'needing people to acknowledge what's going on for you so that they can support you and at the same time feeling isolated because of that or feeling a burden on people'. These conflicting needs can place enormous strains on our intimate relationships and can pose enormous challenges to our self-expression. Negotiating our specific needs such as one's need to rest or have a particular diet can, in this context, be daunting at the very least. Often it may seem easier to not say anything at all, thereby increasing one's sense of isolation and contributing, as Rebecca says, to '... feeling more and more that you are retreating, retreating'.

As well as the difficulties of having to negotiate your particular needs in social situations, there is also the question of feeling apart from the group because of them. I well remember the plight of a mother with a gallstone problem who had to have a special low-fat diet. One of the most devastating things about having her illness was not being able to partake of the same food as the rest of her family each night. The ritual of sharing the meal she had cooked for her family was such a fundamental act of family cohesion and unity for her.

Self-doubt and uncertainty

When confronted with the loss of our identity, our livelihood and important relationships in our lives, the spectres of self-doubt and insecurity can begin to loom large. The experience of illness undoubtedly has brought a lot of uncertainty into the lives of those interviewed. As Rebecca puts it: '... it's not great when you don't know what's going to happen to you and you don't know if it's going to get worse or you're going to be like this for the rest of your life.' Such uncertainty is difficult to live with and can serve to create a separation between the person with illness and the outside world. What is possible in one's life can seem profoundly diminished and at times irretrievably lost.

Many of those interviewed also found the uncertainty in regard to their daily physical symptoms difficult. Kathryn Skelsey recalls feeling really puffed after going up and down stairs and wondering: 'Is this because of the overall illness, or is it that I'm not feeling too well today, or am I getting older, or what is it?' Peter de Reuter recounts the constant struggle involved when getting minor symptoms such as a bruise or some diarrhoea and how easy it is to worry that it might be an AIDS-related illness. Such uncertainty can start to eat away at our self-confidence and further increase our general anxiety levels.

The physical incapacitation that can come with illness can also have profound effects on our emotional wellbeing. This has certainly been the experience of Sara Chesterman who describes how having quadriplegia has made her feel vulnerable physically. Prior to her illness she had had enormous confidence in her physical body and her ability to move around in the world. Sara talks about the emotional repercussions of the loss of her physical mobility and physicality and how differently people walking down the street react to her now that she is in a wheelchair. Her experience of such a basic human interaction had changed fundamentally and profoundly affected her sense of herself in the world.

The challenge to maintain one's self-esteem through the experience of illness is a theme that comes through strongly in the stories of those interviewed. This point is poignantly made by Kathryn Skelsey when she describes how Cushing's disease has increased the roundness of her face, produced more facial hair and thinned the hair on top of her head. These parts of our body are so closely linked to self-esteem for most people. Kathryn also speaks of how the experience of illness made her question her relationship with God. She tells of being very angry with God and resentful at not being helped by him. This led to her rejecting God at times and dramatically affected her relationship with the divine as she understood it.

In the stories of both Sara Chesterman and Peter de Reuter we hear how their experiences of having quadriplegia and being HIV positive have also threatened their sense of themselves as sexual beings, and how challenging this has been for them. As our libidinous energy is so closely aligned with our innate capacity for self-healing, it is easy to see how debilitating this threat to our sexual identity can be.

In this climate one can become extremely sensitive to the reactions of other people to one's situation and for many the easiest way of dealing with this is simply to avoid contact with people. Many of those interviewed describe times during their struggle to regain their health when they preferred to keep their own company. One could also argue that these times were important periods of healing for those interviewed which allowed 'inner work' to take place. By 'inner work' I mean a deeper level of introspection and contemplation than is normally the case for the person concerned. Although immensely challenging, it can also provide a foundation for growth and maturation not otherwise available to the individual. This idea is explored further in later chapters of this book.

On a practical level, healing from a serious illness can be an expensive process and ultimately very draining on one's financial resources. The financial gap between medical specialists' fees and the cover provided by private health insurance can be considerable. Many complementary health care practitioners do not receive any Medicare rebate and often their services are not covered by private health insurance at all. As well, hospital stays and time off work recuperating from surgery or trying to regain one's health can further erode one's financial base. Sadly, the importance of such factors is not always fully appreciated by health care practitioners. In this respect specialist doctors are sometimes the worst offenders, tending to be focused on a specific system of the body. With such a narrow focus, it is easy for the broader social implications of the disease or condition, such as the patient's financial situation, to get lost.

The need for genuine empathy and understanding

One of the things that has struck me during my professional life is how little some doctors actually know about what happens to the lives of their patients once they walk out of their consulting rooms. How people cope financially when they are no longer able to continue their usual work and what happens to their self-esteem when they find themselves at home for long stretches of time are often not considered during the medical consultation. Yet such factors are of vital importance in the journey back to wellbeing and need to be talked about.

In order to understand the reticence of doctors to discuss these issues with their patients I think we need to look at the traditional training of doctors. Medical education up until recent times has focused to a considerable extent on building up technical knowledge of how to treat and diagnose illness. Too often, as the general public often complains, the person with the illness is lost amidst a battery of tests and treatment protocols. Fortunately, in the last twenty years this deficiency in the medical syllabus is starting to be addressed in medical schools as the impact of illness on all different levels of a person's experience is examined.

Over the last ten years I have been fortunate to be involved in one such program. At the University of NSW, the School of Public Health and Community Medicine runs a subject called Introductory Clinical and

Behavioural Studies, which is designed to improve the communication skills of first-year medical students and examines the psychological and social aspects of illness. As part of this course students are required to write a biography, based on six one-hour interviews, of someone who has had a major illness. The interviews focus on how that person coped emotionally, spiritually and financially with the experience of illness. It is hoped that with this broader perspective of illness the doctors of tomorrow will be more able to treat their patients with the respect and humanity they deserve.

In his book *Anatomy of an Illness*, Norman Cousins writes of his own experience of being a patient in hospital and eloquently describes how difficult this time was for him emotionally. He speaks of his 'morbid fear of technology' and his 'strange encounters with compact machines and blinking lights and whirling discs.' In the midst of his feelings of helplessness and apprehension he also speaks of '... the utter void created by the longing – ineradicable, unremitting, pervasive – for the warmth of human contact. A warm smile and an outstretched hand were valued even above the offerings of modern science, but the latter were far more accessible than the former.'

During my own illness, which I speak of in some detail in the chapter entitled 'Physician heal thyself', there was also a time when that sense of warmth and connection was valued above all else. After six months in which dull abdominal pain had become a constant companion, and with it a gnawing feeling of being apart from the rest of the world, to feel another person's warmth and genuine interest offered relief; relief from a private world that was essentially bleak in outlook.

In my visits to different health care practitioners, whether they were complementary or mainstream, I quickly knew whether they really cared about my wellbeing or not. Whatever their knowledge or ability in their chosen field, it soon became apparent if they had my interests at heart, and naturally I responded to their treatments accordingly. These experiences as a patient were also instrumental in enabling me to re-examine the way I had been practising medicine before my illness.

Prior to getting sick, as someone who has always enjoyed good health, there were times when it was hard for me not to feel overwhelmed and sometimes resentful of people's suffering. Generally I felt interested in the experience of my patients, but after ten years in clinical practice including a considerable period counselling people, I started to become more intolerant of my patients. At worst I saw myself as a receptacle for human suffering and would often feel drained at the end of my day's work. I knew that my attitude was part of the problem, yet in the midst of a busy medical practice and my teaching commitments I was at a loss as to how to renew my enthusiasm for my work.

With my experience of being seriously ill with amoebic colitis came a more genuine interest in what my patients were going through and real empathy for their predicaments. My capacity to really be with their struggle had changed markedly. It became possible for me to let go of any judgements that I might previously have had about why they got sick and how they were living their lives. The old adage 'There but for the grace of God go I' was embraced from the heart rather than as something I knew intellectually. The beauty of this transformation in my attitude, apart from the fact that I was now much freer to really be with my patients, was that I was again enjoying my work. I had come to spend a lot of energy protecting myself from my patients in lots of little ways and had become more stingy in how much time I would spend with them. With this change of heart I found myself feeling invigorated by my work and approaching it in a much more relaxed way.

> 'At worst I saw myself as a receptacle for human suffering and would often end up feeling drained and burnt out at the end of my day's work'

Around the time I began to notice these important if somewhat subtle changes, I remember a conversation with Peter de Reuter. As a health care practitioner who has had to live with his own mortality on a daily basis, Peter spoke of how his illness had profoundly affected his ability to feel empathy for his clients. As he put it, there are times when he feels empathy in every tissue of his body for the person in front of him. This joining of the healer and the person coming to be healed is such an important ingredient in the therapeutic encounter.

* * * * * *

In the next chapter I look at the qualities that the individuals interviewed for this book embody and how they have been able to utilise these qualities in their recovery from serious illness.

The road to recovery

'Being sick has forced me on a journey of personal exploration.'
PETER DE REUTER

In reviewing the stories of the people interviewed for this book I have been impressed with how all of them have been able to maximise their natural talents and temperaments in their journeys of healing. Each of them brings to bear their own unique strengths of personality that have allowed them to move beyond the obstacles that lay before them. I would now like to look more closely at how they found their unique roads to recovery.

Harnessing one's inner resources

Sitting with Nicki Youdale I was struck by her natural pragmatism in how she has engineered a program for maintaining wellness. For me this quality stands out in her attitude to her doctors and other health care professionals. She advocates what she calls being 'proactive', asking questions and trying different treatments because, as she puts it, '... at the end of the day no-one really gives a damn about you.' She then wholeheartedly takes up the challenge of getting herself well with the help of various therapists and medical practitioners.

The other qualities I feel Nicki embodies so powerfully are a gritty determination and courage. She says quite frankly that the journey of healing requires a lot of hard work initially and that '... the hard work is bloody hard. It's really scary sometimes and it's really lonely, you get really pissed off.' This sentiment comes through strongly in the stories of several of the people interviewed. Anna also talks of how hard the experience of illness can be and also how interesting it can be at other times. She sees it in terms of an adventure that needs to be fully embraced. In her view, illness needs to be seen as something that life throws at you for really good reasons, an idea that we will explore further in the chapter 'The gift of illness'.

For me the gritty determination that Nicki exudes is evident at the point in her story where she decides to take an active part in her recovery. She tells of doing the 'rounds of naturopaths', seeing a Chinese herbalist and other assorted complementary health practitioners. Despite all her efforts it seemed that none of the treatments was helping her symptoms. At this point it would have been tempting to call it a day and go back to her surgeons. However, Nicki continued to stay open to possible ways to enhance her health and took up the suggestion of someone to see a holistic general practitioner. Nicki was also willing to give his treatment regimen a go, effectively giving her five years of really good health.

In his journey of healing Peter de Reuter brings to bear his keen intellect and powers of discernment. This is particularly evident in how he understands the road to recovery. 'So healing for me is a process whereby I'm using my condition to grow from unconscious levels. It is constantly trying to understand, "What is it that I'm blocking in my life? What is it that I'm not understanding? What am I resisting in my life?" ' For Peter, physical symptoms also have a metaphysical background, which needs to be explored in order for healing to take place. In this way his illness becomes a tool 'to sharpen my knife of consciousness'.

What is so impressive here is Peter's capacity to look at himself with an enormous degree of honesty and his ability to work with what is. In this context he makes the important differentiation between healing and curing; a distinction that, as he says, is often lost in the realms of mainstream medical practice. Generally speaking, the aim in mainstream medical practice is to treat the symptoms and signs of a disease so that the person is free from them or at least able to successfully manage them so there is minimal interference in their daily life. However, as Peter points out, what is important in his experience is how much healing has happened along the way; healing being a process whereby there is a fundamental reorganisation of our being, a process that brings us in the direction of greater balance and harmony.

In this context healing may involve working through emotional scars from the past or transforming limiting attitudes about life that have never previously been questioned. Thus illness can become the catalyst for change at the very deepest levels of our being. As Peter goes on to say: 'I may die from this condition but that doesn't mean that I have failed.'

By way of contrast, Anna River's approach to her recovery relied more on her intuition about what she needed to do to heal herself. She describes approaching her t'ai chi teacher wanting to learn how to meditate. When questioned by him as to why she wanted to meditate, she replied, 'Why not?' But as she goes on to say, '... I thought about it, "I don't know why I want to do this thing." ' Rather than researching on the Internet, or systematically seeking out the opinions of health care experts, Anna would naively be drawn to those practices and healing traditions that her healing required. At different times in her recovery, relying on this inner knowing, Anna took up meditation, spinning wool and writing to herself.

In keeping with this more organic approach to her own healing is her innate sensibility about what she could and couldn't do at different stages in her recovery. She describes how she realised that for a long time after doing her initial Vipassana meditation course she was too unsettled and agitated to meditate at home. Many people faced with this experience might come to the conclusion that meditation is not for them. But Anna in her wisdom wasn't prepared to force herself and realised that her meditation practice at home would 'fall into place when it was meant to', rather than imposing a discipline on herself which would be bound to fail. Her story is a profound illustration of the beauty of allowing the process of healing to unfold in its own time for, as she says, '... the organism itself knows when it's ready for certain things.'

Sara Chesterman's strongly positive frame of thinking is clearly evident in the first sentence of her interview with me when she describes her quadriplegia in this way: '... I have full function in my body from the neck up and I've got full arm function apart from my fingers (which I can't move at all) ...' What is emphasised is what she does have rather than focusing on what she doesn't have. For Sara the glass is half full rather than half empty. Implicit in her view of her situation is her capacity to be philosophical about the situation she has found herself in. This is particularly evident in how she has managed to see the brighter side of her disability and how she has been able to work with it. She recounts how threatened she initially felt by the looks on people's faces in the street when they saw her in her wheelchair and how she has been able to turn those feelings around. She talks about how she is now in a more powerful position to make an impact on people and in some instances to help them feel more comfortable with disability by simply being more relaxed in herself. She even concludes that given her character she is 'quite suited to being in a wheelchair'. One cannot help but be moved by her lightness and humour.

> 'I may die from this condition but that doesn't mean I have failed'

Hand in hand with Sara's quality of lightness is her natural creativity, which she has brought to bear in her approach to her disability. Her love of dancing and movement has been taken to new levels through the experience of quadriplegia and led her to a deeper understanding of what her passion for dance was about. '... it's about interacting with other people and seeing how different bodies move.' She goes on to describe seeing an able-bodied woman and a woman with paraplegia dancing together and the inherent beauty of them both. One gets the impression from listening to Sara that her condition has served to open more doors for her to the wonder and awe of living.

The courage to embrace change

One of the traits that characterises most, if not all, of those interviewed is a willingness to embrace new and often confronting levels of experience. Rather than staying with the inherent limitations of the situation in which they found themselves, the individuals in this book have stepped beyond their comfort zones and opened themselves to the unknown. This willingness, which could also be termed courage, is typified in the story of Janelle Meisner who tried many different psychotherapeutic approaches to help her deal with her panic attacks and post-traumatic stress disorder. She recounts her ongoing fragility while having somatic psychotherapy and the life-changing insights she had when later studying this body-oriented approach to understanding human experience. 'I realised ... that I didn't understand a lot of things. I had lived my life thinking that it was normal to be cold; it was normal to be in a sweat and cold at the same time. Things like that were just normal to me.' Through a comprehensive re-examination of how she had been operating in the world, and with the guidance of some wise and skilled teachers, Janelle was able to move towards better health and new levels of personal wellbeing.

Another quality that Janelle embodies is that capacity to do whatever it takes to get well, despite the cost to other people's or society's perception of her. In pursuing the circuitous path to better health, Janelle was willing to use all her available resources; in her case this meant selling her business and using up her savings. This stands in direct contrast to what I have observed in other people in my medical practice, who when faced with potentially life-threatening illness seem intent on maintaining their six-figure incomes and expensive lifestyles rather than devote more energy to their own healing. Janelle's ability to let go of her pride is also apparent in how she was able to change the way she had been practising yoga. Prior to her illness, her yoga practice had been ruled by a need to do her yoga postures perfectly, she had to get them right! Letting go, into what for her felt like a 'sloppy' yoga practice, was a huge achievement which no doubt helped to loosen the perfectionism that was underpinning her approach to living.

Deep and honest self-examination

Another factor that seems to me to be central to the process of recovery, which is evident in all of those interviewed, is a capacity for deep introspection coupled with an ability to make changes to their view of themselves and lifestyles. In this sense, Kathryn Skelsey's experience of illness forced her into a more mature examination of herself and why she got sick as well as her relationship with God. She talks of the 'uncomfortable process of going into really dark spaces' that she would have preferred not to have ventured into. She doesn't profess to know why she had to go down that path but has come to some kind of acceptance of life's ups and downs. Along the way Kathryn has got some acute insights into the nature of healing and she has been quick to try a number of different approaches to facilitate her return to wellness.

Using her common sense and initiative, Kathryn was quick to take control of her situation and worked out her own therapeutic approach to getting well. This included a basic approach to diet, improving her circulation as a means of clearing her body of excess hormones, practising self-massage and breathing practices and doing things she really enjoys like dancing and painting. Another aspect of her therapy was to search out and spend more time with people she likes and who respond positively to her. Having such supportive social environments has helped her to move through negative states of mind and allowed her to trust other people more.

Rebecca Hutchinson in her struggle to overcome chronic fatigue syndrome also displays this capacity for rigorous self-examination. Her perceptions about how she became sick and how the experience of illness has afforded her opportunities for spiritual growth are certainly remarkable. Throughout her interview Rebecca eloquently describes her understanding of why she got sick, how the experience of illness has affected her and what she has learnt about herself along the way. Illness has been a profoundly humbling experience for her, and as she says, '... it's a good thing to realise you're human ...'. Rebecca goes on to say how being sick has made her more able to be truly empathetic with other people's suffering and profoundly changed her view around what it means to be vulnerable.

What comes through so strongly in Rebecca's words is her ability to stay with the big picture, despite the obvious hardships she has been suffering, and to see the humourous side to her struggle. She talks of longing for a quiet life during her university days, when she was desperately trying to prove herself to the world, but of not having the personal resources to get her to that place. Ultimately it was only through illness that she was able to manifest a quiet life as a yoga teacher. As she goes on to joke, 'Try another route next time!' But as she is quick to point out, for her there was no other way because '... you have to break. The ego has to crumble, which it did.'

Harnessing the power within

The ability to harness and successfully utilise one's willpower is clearly evident in the story of Shankardev Saraswati's struggle to overcome asthma. Shankardev is blessed with, by his own admission, a tenacious character. Once he had decided yoga was the path for him he simply put his mind to follow it assiduously. In his case this meant travelling to India to undergo intensive yogic training. I understand, though it was not mentioned in his interview, that his guru's ashram is located in the middle of Bihar, a state of India infamous for its lawlessness and poverty. The very act of travelling to the ashram by himself from Australia and overcoming the fears inherent in such a journey shows considerable determination and strength of character.

Coupled with Shankardev's tremendous tenacity of purpose is his capacity for self-discipline. Prior to his breakthrough experience, while lying sick in bed in the ashram in India, which signalled the end of his asthma, Shankardev had been practising various yoga postures, breathing exercises and meditation and cleansing practices for two years. He had then undertaken a more intensive set of yogic practices, which took three hours a day while living a spartan life in the setting of his guru's ashram. While this level of discipline is probably well beyond many people and may not be the path that is necessarily right for them, it has clearly brought great benefits for Shankardev. It was during this disciplined exploration of yogic practices that he had what he described as '... a vision of what yoga potentially could do but also how much was required to get to that depth [of healing].' Thus his ability to discipline himself and follow the guidance of his guru brought insights into himself that paved the way for the healing he so desperately sought; the healing not only of his asthma but also of the emotional turmoil and pain that he had been experiencing at that time in his life.

* * * * * *

Having looked at the various qualities that the individuals interviewed for this book embody and which have taken them on their journeys of healing thus far, in the next chapter I would like to turn our attention to what they have learnt along the way.

Healing as learning

> 'The journey of healing, if it's a worthwhile and real healing, I think is definitely a journey of learning. It's learning about the world and other people, but it's really learning about yourself.'
> ANNA RIVERS

I would now like to focus on what the individuals interviewed for this book have learnt from their experience of being sick. That illness can be a profound catalyst for learning is an idea not often embraced in the world at large. More often illness is viewed in negative terms and sometimes seen as the result of 'bad karma' or sins one has committed previously in one's life; something to be got rid of and amputated from one's life. That illness is a valid experience, as valid as any other, a point made by Shankardev Saraswati in his interview, is too often lost in modern Western culture with its preoccupation with glamorous physical health and beauty. Readily apparent in the stories of the eight individuals interviewed, however, is the sense of illness providing opportunities for learning profound lessons about the process of living. These opportunities might otherwise be denied us, if not for the experience of serious illness.

Several of them describe the process of learning about their bodies and how this has been an integral part of their experience of healing. Janelle Meisner, in her battle with chronic fatigue syndrome, underwent what she describes as an 'incredible exploratory journey inside my body'. By seeing a somatic or body-oriented psychotherapist and undergoing training in this field she went through a profound re-experiencing of her body. Through this work she realised that chronic fatigue syndrome was 'a lifetime of having nowhere to rest'. Prior to her illness she had never learnt how to find a place of rest inside herself.

Here Janelle is using the word 'rest' in a particular way and it is perhaps useful to say a little about what I think she means. 'Rest' in this context is a state of quite deep relaxation of the body and mind which many people rarely experience in their everyday lives. When the bodymind is chronically running in overdrive, with lots of adrenaline being produced, true rest is not possible and one's whole system tends to get depleted of available energy. What she is referring to here is having times in one's life when one's whole system can really let go; for some of us this may come a few weeks into a very relaxing holiday or at the end of a really good massage from our favourite masseur. It is also true that some people have learned to live their lives in a basically relaxed fashion, in tune with their bodies and feelings, and so have ample periods to rest and have people who they can rest into when the going gets tough.

Later in her interview Janelle goes on to talk about learning to self-regulate; in simple terms, how to really listen to your body and be attentive to its (your) needs. Self-regulation requires you to be sensitive to signals from your body that tell you you are going beyond your limits and respond to these cues in ways that honour the body's needs at that moment. For Janelle, this process was also helped by learning a style of yoga that encouraged her to stay within her limits and not to push her body. Unfortunately, not all yoga teachers or even schools of yoga adhere to these principles of respect for one's body, which seems contrary to the spirit of yoga.

Rebecca Hutchinson takes up this point, too, emphasising the importance of honouring the body and listening to it because, as she says, 'It's the one that really knows.' Most of us tend to relate to our bodily symptoms as a nuisance or even a curse rather than acknowledging that they are giving us important information that we can utilise in getting ourselves back into balance. All too often we have some rigid notion of what we should be able to do, which is totally out of relationship with the actual reality of how our body feels. In this context it is easy to feel let down by our body rather than have a more accepting view of ourselves. This notion that there is an inherent link between our physical symptoms and our mental and emotional life is explored further in the chapter on bodymind healing.

As a sufferer of thalidomide-induced heart disease, Nicki Youdale has known breathlessness most of her life. In searching for ways to improve her respiratory capacity and improve her breathing she came across the Buteyko method. Using this breathing technique she has been able to profoundly improve her energy levels, sleep and circulation. Rebecca Hutchinson also describes the benefits of learning how to breath better through doing specifically tailored yogic breathing practices taught to her by a medical doctor who is also a trained yoga therapist. The acquisition of a new skill, in this case something seemingly so basic as learning how to breathe properly, helped her to make a real difference to her recovery. To be able to simply and without anyone else's help make ourselves feel better no doubt has a very positive effect on our self-esteem. It is often easy to feel disempowered and helpless when we are dependent on others to get relief from our suffering.

'Chronic fatigue syndrome was "a lifetime of having nowhere to rest"'

Anna Rivers applied herself over many years to the task of mastering a meditation practice. In her battle to repair the 'rent in the fabric' of her mind, after suffering a psychotic episode over several months that left her profoundly debilitated, Anna learnt Vipassana meditation. She even describes this approach to meditation as the most important part of her healing because it helped her to integrate some of the experiences she had during her period of madness into the rest of her life. Anna explains how Vipassana meditation – a Buddhist meditation practice brought to the West by a Burmese man, S. N. Goenka – was able to help her release a lot of 'stuck' negative emotions. With this gradual transformation she was able to get out of her head, where she had been living a lot of the time, and be more in the moment. No longer caught up in thought patterns based in her past, Anna's sleep improved dramatically, as did her clarity of thought. The meditation practice had the effect of giving her some mental distance from her 'particular brand of psychotic thinking', thus paving the way for her rehabilitation and recovery from mental illness.

The benefit of learning meditation also comes through in the experience of Rebecca Hutchinson who, with the guidance of a yoga teacher, established a meditation practice that has become a part of her daily routine. In her case she drew sustenance also from a spiritual teaching called Vedanta, which sees our essential nature as timeless and formless. It teaches that we are not our bodies, which, as Rebecca describes, was a really liberating thought for her, helping her to see beyond the limitations of her condition and to embrace her illness as her teacher. Janelle Meisner also learnt how to meditate, in her case using different Buddhist practices that suited her temperament and the nature of her condition. She talks of doing little bits of meditation often, rather than the more orthodox approach of having to sit for long periods of time in order to get any benefit.

The individuality of each person's approach to their own healing is a point emphasised by a number of the people interviewed. Rebecca puts it neatly, 'As our nature is individual, so is our healing.' She goes on to advocate, for people actively involved in their own recovery, the importance of searching for and learning about 'things that resonate deeply with your being' in order to support the process of healing.

Illness as a teacher

Inherent in the stories of all eight individuals is a strong sense of how the experience of illness has facilitated their understanding of themselves as human beings. What is intriguing is: how was this process of self-exploration supported for these individuals? Janelle Meisner likens her experience of illness to having a very long retreat after which 'I came out knowing much better who I was and what was important, and who my friends actually were.' She is in no doubt that there was an emotional base to her chronic fatigue syndrome and post-traumatic stress disorder and received considerable help from various forms of psychotherapy. She also recounts trying many forms of bodywork, not always with positive results. Though, in the final analysis, it was while having bodywork that she experienced a profound turning point in her illness. This occurred during a bodywork session when she experienced at a deep level being totally acknowledged and accepted by another human being, through the medium of touch. The very possibility of this connection melted years of distrust and self-imposed isolation.

This theme of illness as a vehicle for self-knowledge is taken up in the story of Rebecca Hutchinson who benefited enormously from two years of psychotherapy with a doctor and yoga therapist. Her therapy included a grounding in yogic philosophy, and Ayurveda helped her come to terms with what was happening in her life, and more specifically, how to be with it. In both her story and that of Janelle Meisner, the sense of shame they experienced about being sick comes through quite palpably. Sufferers of chronic fatigue syndrome were, and still are, often considered malingerers; the general reception of other people to their plight is not always supportive.

Anna Rivers in her interview echoes many of these sentiments. She describes how difficult it was having to face the judgements of friends; friends who were unable to acknowledge the immensity of her experience, and labelled it as simply a drug-induced psychosis. So initially Anna withdrew from social interactions, but later in her journey she realised how important it was for her to express herself more fully in her relationship with other human beings. She says: 'I'd reached that point of healing where I felt that in order for anyone to know me, I had to say, "Look, I'm just not an ordinary person, I've had this thing happen. But it's alright. It's okay." ' And so from that point onwards she tentatively started to open up to those people whom she felt safe with, whom she determined would not judge her experience but be interested and actually listen to her.

The power of expressing ourselves and giving vent to our deepest feelings is also taken up in the experience of Nicki Youdale in her battle with major heart and respiratory disease. During her long experience of illness Nicki has learnt the value of finding people with whom we can express ourselves freely. Her message to other sufferers of illness is very clear: 'If you have trouble dealing with certain things about health or whatever, don't keep it to yourself. Go and talk to professionals and shop around until you find the best psychologist, psychiatrist, friend, whatever. Don't keep it to yourself. Everything is much better out than in, don't store the tears up ... Just get it out ...' For many of us the ability to express our deepest feelings is not something that comes easily, often because of fear of judgement or being shamed we will endure anything rather than expose ourselves to such a potentially hurtful experience. In this context, the experience of really being listened to by another human being and not judged is profoundly healing. Moreover, such an experience gives tacit encouragement that there are people out there who are not interested in dismissing our experience but in valuing it.

Finding and accepting support

Another skill learnt by some of the individuals interviewed is the ability to know where to find support and to be able to reach out and accept that support. Often there is a sense that somehow we should be able to deal with whatever challenges life presents us with. However, when we are faced with a situation, such as a major illness, that we may not have the skills to deal with, it is a powerful opportunity to learn from others. In her struggle with Cushing's disease, Kathryn Skelsey talks of actively searching out people she likes and consciously trying to spend more time with them. Through being with people who respond positively to her she is able to re-experience herself and, as she says, this has helped her to trust in people more.

The importance of having people around you who are able to support you when you are at your most vulnerable is a theme that emerges from the experience of those interviewed. The acceptance offered by those people nurtures one's self-esteem and challenges any sense one might have of feeling a failure for getting sick in the first place.

We can see in the stories of those interviewed that they have all learnt some important lessons as a result of their experience of serious illness; lessons that have given them a stronger sense of themselves as individuals in the world and which helped them recover their health and sense of wellbeing. One gets the definite feeling that these eight people now have a more solid grasp of who they are and what is important to them in their lives. This is a point that I would like to examine more closely as it seems to me that it is no coincidence that such an existential journey has gone hand in hand with improvement in their physical health. Indeed, this correlation is completely in line with the principles of healing described in Ayurveda.

The benefit of following your unique *dharma*

Ayurveda, the traditional system of medicine in India and a science focused on the treatment of disease, is also concerned with how best to preserve one's health and wellbeing. As a science it seeks to help people attain four principal aims of life. As described in Ayurveda, these aims are *dharma*, *artha*, *kama* and *moksha*. These are all words in Sanskrit, the language of ancient India, and although these words have no simple English translation, I will endeavour to give you a sense of how they can be understood in a contemporary setting.

> '... a situation – such as a major illness – that we may not have the skills to deal with, [offers] a powerful opportunity to learn from others'

Of these four aims I am going to concentrate mainly on the concept of *dharma* because it is particularly relevant to my understanding of why the individuals in this book have been able to bring about the healing they have achieved. *Dharma* is the first of the four aims and is a complex concept, which has been interpreted in different ways through the ages. When used at the level of the individual, it refers to that path through life that allows a person to achieve their full potential and to fulfil their own unique destiny. One's *dharma* is a calling to honour and actualise one's uniqueness as a human being. It is not a selfish endeavour but rather something that will 'carry' one through one's life. Honouring our *dharma* may involve doing things that are boring, inconvenient and even painful; however, living in accordance with our *dharma* is innately satisfying at a deep level. Our *dharma* not only contributes to our own personal wellbeing, it also is beneficial for our families and communities.

In my own case, an aspect of my *dharma* has been to teach and practise Ayurvedic medicine in the West. Along the way I have been privileged to meet with a wonderful array of students; some of these students have also gone on to teach and practise Ayurveda. The friendships that have developed as a result of my commitment to Ayurveda have been a rich source of satisfaction and support for me. This commitment to Ayurveda has also moved me to study its sister sciences – yoga, Vedic astrology and Vedic architecture. The knowledge and understanding I have received from these traditions has further enriched my life as well as the lives of my family, friends and the students.

As part of my exploration of Ayurveda I have studied Ayurvedic massage, which uses oils medicated with various herbs according to time-honoured traditions. I have also received different types of Ayurvedic massage that, apart from being very rejuvenating and beneficial for my health, have encouraged me to establish my own self-massage regimen on a daily basis. When I became a father I was naturally keen to share my enjoyment of massage with my son, which became a wonderful time of bonding for us both. It was also a great way to help soothe his nervous system and was very useful in the treatment of the colic he experienced from time to time. In these ways, through following my *dharma* I have been profoundly nourished and supported. Ayurveda has thus been a powerful vehicle that has carried me through my life.

For some people it may be their *dharma* to devote themselves to motherhood, for others it may be through being a musician or a shopkeeper. What matters, it would seem, is the deep sense of satisfaction that we derive from what it is we do. In this way our *dharma* has a protective function in our journey through life and brings a sense of knowing that this is the life we were born into. Our *dharma* enables us to find out where our own individual thread fits into the overall tapestry of life.

The concept of *dharma* as a way of living that nourishes our souls and sustains our families and communities is central to Ayurveda's approach to supporting one's health. When we are living in tune with our *dharma*, our life force – called *prana* in yoga and *qi* in Traditional Chinese Medicine – is immeasurably stronger. We feel more energised, our physical health is naturally more robust and our capacity to enjoy life is greater. By way of contrast, living out of alignment with our *dharma* will make life more difficult for us as individuals. Our physical health is more likely to suffer, our moods will be more unstable and our sense of wellbeing diminished. Most of us have experienced times in our lives when some activity we were involved in brought with it deep levels of satisfaction; that sense of, 'This is what I'm meant to be doing!' This may involve considerable effort and struggle, but at the end of the day such activity brings with it a stronger sense of one's place in the universe.

Earlier in my medical career, I remember seeing a young man in his early twenties who was referred to me because of disillusionment and mild depression. Joshua's father had died a year previously and his mother had strongly encouraged him to join a prominent banking institution, where he was working as a clerk. When we first met he had a negative and cynical view of life. His world had become innately dissatisfying. During our talks it emerged that his real passion in life was acting. However, his mother had strongly discouraged him from following what seemed to her a difficult and unreliable career path. Joshua, with my support, applied to a number of acting schools and was later accepted into one of the most prestigious acting schools in the country. When I saw him several years later he was working in Sydney with a successful acting troupe doing Shakespearian comedies. His posture and demeanour had totally changed; he exuded a confidence and enthusiasm that was infectious and was obviously thriving in the creative milieu that acting provided for him. I had a strong sense that Joshua was living in line with his *dharma*; needless to say my counselling services were no longer necessary.

For all of those interviewed for this book one gets a strong sense that their healing journey has brought with it profound changes in how they view themselves and the world around them. Some have changed their livelihoods, others have not, but for all of them there have been important internal shifts in how they are going about the process of living their lives. These shifts have entailed critical re-examination of core beliefs and attitudes and have facilitated personal growth and a more authentic level of self-expression. As they have moved to fulfil their unique *dharmas* their wellbeing – at the physical, emotional, mental and spiritual levels – has followed.

The second aim of life in Ayurveda, *artha*, relates to the pursuit of security, which may be through gathering wealth, power and/or fame. It is also the means by which we are able to support ourselves in our journey through life. *Kama*, the third aim of life in Ayurveda, relates to the pursuit of pleasure, in the form of simple desires such as the wish to enjoy your children, a beautiful piece of music or the warmth of the sun's rays on your back. The fourth aim of life in the Ayurvedic world-view is *moksha*, which means 'liberation'. It relates to the spiritual domain of our lives and is concerned with such questions as 'Who am I?' and 'What will happen to me when I die?' It involves coming to terms in a meaningful way with the transitory nature of our lives on this planet.

The Ayurvedic paradigm thus views health in the broadest possible way, with the treatment of physical disease being only a part of its general scope. As a model of health it affirms to a remarkable extent the experience of the eight people interviewed for this book and how they understand the healing process. We will explore this theme further in the next chapter.

Healing the whole person

'According to my personal experience, mental stability and physical wellbeing are directly related. Without question, anger and agitation make us more susceptible to illness. On the other hand, if the mind is tranquil and occupied with positive thoughts, the body will not easily fall prey to disease.'
TENZIN GYATSO, THE 14TH DALAI LAMA

I thought it appropriate to begin this chapter with this quote from the Dalai Lama for several reasons. The Dalai Lama, like the individuals interviewed, speaks from his own experience and, like many of the individuals interviewed for this book, acknowledges the profound connection between the mind and the body. The idea that what we think and feel as human beings can influence the state of our physical health is certainly not new. Indeed it is part and parcel of how most, if not all, indigenous systems of medicine understand health and disease. Later in this chapter we will see how the ancient Indian tradition of yoga conceives the human being and its different layers, and how this understanding influences the yogic approach to healing. For now I would like to come back to the experience of those interviewed for this book.

Rebecca Hutchinson has no doubt that the cause of her chronic fatigue syndrome was related to some underlying attitudes that were driving her behaviour. '... I think I had some pretty strong patterns of behaviour and thinking, things that were really weakening my immune system.' She is now able to identify the rising anxiety that in the past drove her to get really busy in her life and to go beyond the limits of her body. This process she now realises has had a very depleting effect on her body and has led to profound states of exhaustion. As a result of the experience of illness Rebecca can now see how these tendencies put enormous pressure on her immune system. She knows that how she has been emotionally in the world has exacerbated her immune system problem to breaking point, thereby paving the way for her illness to manifest itself.

While acknowledging the role played by a constitutional weakness and dietary factors in making him more prone to having asthma as a child, Shankardev Saraswati speaks of the impact of psychological stresses in causing his condition, his parents having both been traumatised by the horrors of living through World War II in Europe. The emotional climate in the family home was obviously a difficult one and as he says: 'So my asthma attacks were a way of getting some emotional support.' He later goes on to speak of the profound healing of his asthma that came with a deep understanding of how he was holding himself as a person, while undergoing intensive yogic practices in India. A shift in his body took place in tandem with a shift in self-understanding. For Shankardev, the innate influence of the mind on the body and the body on the mind is clear.

In her battle with Cushing's disease, Kathryn Skelsey also speaks of the link between her mind and her physical health. As she recounts: 'I think the trigger for my relapse the second time round was another relationship situation.' She goes on to describe being worn down by a long-distance relationship and feeling emotionally torn as to whether she should continue in this relationship. Her quandary was exacerbated by her high ideals about what sort of person her life partner should be and her personal misgivings about the man she was in relationship with.

Inherent in the stories of many of those interviewed is the theme that their illness arose during a time in their life when there was significant mental and emotional disharmony. The process of their healing enabled them to see just how this disharmony contributed to their illness. It would also seem that this healing process involved a good deal of soul-searching and self-examination. In order to identify the psychological factors that had a bearing on their illness, many of the individuals in this book have entered into counselling and psychotherapy. Armed with insights into themselves derived from these inner journeys, they have then been able to transform their mental and emotional life and thus facilitate the healing of their physical condition. I would now like to look at the basic elements of their approaches to their healing.

The four quadrants of healing

The process of healing is in my experience a complex phenomenon and, as Anna Rivers suggests, multifaceted. In coming to grips with how it occurs Anna talks about healing at four primary levels – the physical, the emotional, the mental and the spiritual levels. I first heard of this approach to understanding healing in the 1980s, from the experience of Dr Elisabeth Kübler-Ross and her work with dying patients. I find it a simple and useful model in understanding the different requirements we as human beings have in order to live satisfying and health-giving lives. Anna brings her own unique perspectives to this model based on her own experience of healing from a psychotic breakdown, perspectives which are eminently practical and bear the stamp of authenticity. But first let us be quite clear about what is meant by these four different quadrants or levels of healing.

> 'She [can] now identify the rising anxiety that in the past drove her to get really busy and to go beyond the limits of her body'

The physical

The physical quadrant of healing, as I understand it, refers to food, exercise and sleep, the three traditional pillars of healthy living. The quality of the food we ingest and how we eat it are basic to how we support the tissues of our bodies. Health-inducing supplements to our diet, such as herbs and vitamins, I would also include under the physical quadrant. Regular exercise, appropriate for our age and condition, whether it be in the form of sporting activities, gym exercises or walking, helps the circulation of fluids around the body and aids digestion. Under exercise we could also include massage as a potent way of revitalising the body and relieving muscular tension. The quality and quantity of sleep we get also has profound implications for our health; adequate, good quality sleep rejuvenates the body and mind on a daily basis.

The emotional

The emotional quadrant of healing is closely connected to the mental quadrant and they are sometimes difficult to differentiate. Emotional healing, in my view, relates to the process whereby we feel more and more comfortable in sharing with others the full range of our feelings. For some this might mean being able to express one's hurt and anger at perceived injustices in one's life, for others it might mean feeling safe enough to allow one's grief to surface from losses experienced in the process of living. Generally, emotional healing relates to being able to express one's deepest feelings with other human beings, rather than becoming more and more isolated. In my professional experience a lot of people when faced with a major illness will find themselves feeling alone and needing support at some point. Rebecca Hutchinson talks candidly about the surge of emotions that come when she is feeling vulnerable: 'That whole fear and sadness of not knowing what's happening and not being able to have power and to be able to cope in life.'

Sometimes the sympathetic ear of a good friend will help see us through these difficult times, though for many this may not be an option for various reasons. As Nicki Youdale clearly states: 'Don't keep it to yourself. Everything is much better out than in, don't store the tears up, don't store the anger up, don't store the fear up. Just get it out ...' Unfortunately, for a lot of people it is not easy advice to follow. This is where seeing a well-trained counsellor or psychotherapist can be extremely helpful. Finding a place in your life where you feel safe to express your most intimate fears and concerns can be a profoundly healing experience.

The mental

The mental quadrant of healing seems to be related to the healing of core belief systems that we live out of and which have a strong effect on how we operate in the world. Often there is little conscious awareness of how these attitudes determine how we react to different types of people and situations. Sara Chesterman talks about how having a disability such as quadriplegia has been a huge threat to her self-esteem. Losing her sense of herself as a sexual being was very difficult, as was having to readjust her basic expectations about what sort of life she could have. Coming from a privileged background, it was natural for Sara to believe that a glamorous and affluent life would always be there for her. After her accident Sara, with the help of a psychologist, was able to examine a lot of her core values and to find new sources of strength in herself.

In her journey towards wellness, Rebecca Hutchinson came to identify patterns in her behaviour based around maintaining robustness and being perceived by the world at large as someone who is strong. Ironically, it was these belief systems that were actually weakening her physical health. She describes early in her interview how at one point in her struggle with chronic fatigue syndrome she would need to lie down on Saturday afternoons. In her world this was not something you did. She had a set of standards about how one should live one's life, which were directly confronted as a result of her illness; standards that ultimately had to be reassessed. In the final analysis her illness came to grant her a licence to live in a more flexible and creative way; a way that ultimately would restore her to much better health, in the fullest sense of the word.

In similar fashion Kathryn Skelsey came to understand patterns in her behaviour that were fundamentally undermining her health. In her case she came to see how her inherent perfectionism had driven her study through high school and her final exams and worn down her immune system, making her more susceptible to getting a major illness. This theme again emerges in the experience of Janelle Meisner who talks of how a strong tendency towards perfectionism played itself out in her approach to living prior to her illness. An example she gives is her approach to doing yoga postures before she became ill: 'If I was going to do it, I was going to do it right!' She was also a very strict vegetarian and as a result of her diet had become underweight. Thus in order for her to balance these strong forces in her psyche, Janelle had to learn how to practise yoga in a more relaxed way – letting go of her need to do the postures perfectly – and how to let go of her attachment to not eating meat.

Janelle's story also highlights another aspect of healing in the mental quadrant; an aspect not often focused on in mainstream medical practice.

For her, part of the process of healing was finding a source of joy and getting her sense of humour back. In order for that to happen she talks of letting go of the story about why you got sick. At this point a word of explanation is timely. 'The story' as I understand it is an attitude towards how you got sick; an attitude that attributes your suffering to some outside agent. It may be that you feel you got sick because you were harassed by your partner or unfairly treated by your employer or by one of your parents. The essence of 'the story' is that somehow you got sick because of someone else. If only my husband hadn't cheated on me, if only my father had been there for me. It keeps you feeling powerless and sees you as the victim in the whole affair of being sick. As Janelle points out, 'people do it differently'.

For her, this is a phenomenon of the bodymind. Having insight into the story is not enough. For healing to occur she says we need to find where the story is trapped in the tissues of our bodies, and work with all its different layers. Janelle here is talking of identifying the attitudes held energetically in the tissues of the body with the aid of somatic or body-oriented psychotherapy and bodywork. Then, through regular sessions with a therapist over months to years, working to regain aliveness in those tissues and thus letting go of the power the story has over you. For those readers not familiar with this field of healing I refer you to the works of Alexander Lowen and Stanley Keleman in the 'Further reading' section at the end of this book.

The spiritual

The spiritual quadrant of healing, by contrast, relates to coming to terms with such basic questions as: What will happen to me when I die? Where was I before I was born? How should I live my life so that on my last sigh I will feel replete? Nicki Youdale's experience of living with heart disease helps shed light on what is meant by healing at this level. She talks of getting to 'a space where you feel more at ease about your mortality' and the freedom and humour that comes with that. For Nicki, it has meant not being so obsessed about the silly little things in life and keeping up appearances. As a result of her experience of illness she has been able to engage with other people in a more direct and honest way. Nicki's story of the time she spent with the young Aboriginal girl in the cardiac ward exemplifies her down to earth and non-judgemental attitude to life.

During his struggle to live with the uncertainties of being HIV positive Peter de Reuter has developed his own particular approach to staying centred. This involves using the present moment as his mantra or focusing point. Thus he is able to bring his practice of meditation into his daily life. 'As much as I can (and I fail miserably most of the time), I try to be in this moment. What am I feeling? What games am I playing? What patterns am I running off? What sort of destructive things or thoughts am I self-talking?' Once he becomes aware of these concerns he then has a choice of whether to give them more energy or to do it differently. Thus through developing this witnessing state in his life Peter endeavours to stay present to each and every moment of his life as best he can, rather than living out of the tyranny of the past. This kind of approach to healing of the spiritual quadrant is mirrored in the experience of Janelle Meisner.

When she found herself not coping with her immediate situation, Janelle tried to notice simply that she was not coping. Rather than castigate herself for not coping, Janelle comes back to the present moment. 'In this moment I'm not coping and that is okay.' Knowing too that this moment will pass she is more able to be with what comes along rather than go down the path of self-recrimination and self-criticism. This process of becoming more mindful, a Buddhist practice, has been accelerated in a very real way through the experience of illness. However, as Janelle has come to realise, there are always more layers of understanding about being mindful. This mental technique that she has used to stay sane during her illness has, as she says, a much broader scope. Indeed, it can be a powerful spiritual practice helping one to live one's life in a meaningful and satisfying way.

The idea that the experience of illness can offer us the opportunity of profound personal transformation comes through strongly in the interview with Rebecca Hutchinson. Prior to her getting chronic fatigue syndrome, Rebecca had a busy life as a university student, struggling to prove herself and yet also yearning to be living a quiet and more spiritual life. She describes going up to the mountains on the weekends and feeling a sadness in herself: '... a longing for something that the mountains embodied. I think now that what they embodied was "being". It felt like things just *were*, and I think I *wasn't*.' Rebecca tells us how illness enabled her to enter a world she could never quite reach before; a world that, prior to getting sick, she did not have the resources within herself to manifest. At the time of the interview with Rebecca she was living a quiet life in the mountains outside Sydney and working as a yoga teacher.

At this point, having reviewed the basic holistic framework inherent in the approaches to healing of the eight people interviewed, I would like to look at an understanding of the human being informed by the ancient healing tradition of yoga. This tradition recognises the intimate connection between the different aspects of human life and sees the human being as a mind–body–spirit complex.

How yoga understands the process of healing

Yoga, the vast spiritual science that originated in the Indian subcontintent thousands of years ago, is concerned with healing of the bodymind. It is derived from the root *yuj* in the Sanskrit language, which means 'to yoke or harness', and is concerned with the question of how to 'yoke' oneself to the divine. It comprises various spiritual disciplines that are aids for those in the quest for enlightenment. In this approach the body and mind are held to be intricately related; as such, yogic practices work equally with both, and physical and breathing practices are prescribed along with mental practices such as meditation.

The principles of yoga can also be utilised in the healing of physical disease, a field of practice known as yoga therapy. Yoga therapy is generally practised by qualified health care practitioners such as doctors, nurses and naturopaths who have also trained in yoga and its application in the treatment of disease. It is an area of endeavour that has only recently begun to receive attention in the West but has long been an aspect of yogic science in India.

Within the world-view of yoga, which is based on the subjective experience in meditation of yogis over thousands of years, the physical body is only one vehicle for the expression of consciousness. The human being is conceived as being composed of five sheaths, much like the concentric layers of an onion. These sheaths are said to be generated as consciousness descends into denser and denser matter. Each sheath provides a platform for the expression of consciousness at that level. Subtler sheaths act as blueprints for the grosser sheaths, with each level of organisation building on the previous one. The five sheaths are called *koshas* in Sanskrit and give us an elegant and comprehensive way of understanding the human being in health and disease. In this view, physical symptoms can sometimes be related to disharmony at deeper levels of our being. The five sheaths are traditionally described in the following way.

1. The *anna-maya-kosha* or literally 'the sheath composed of food' is the most gross physical sheath. It is nourished by the juices extracted from our food and corresponds to the physical body.
2. The *prana-maya-kosha* or literally 'the sheath composed of life force' is said to connect the sheaths of food and the mind and is nourished by *prana*. *Prana* can be translated as our life force and will be better known to some readers by the equivalent term in Traditional Chinese Medicine, *qi*. Our *prana* is an energy that is replenished primarily in two ways, from breathing air and from digesting food in the gut.
3. The *mano-maya-kosha* or literally the 'the sheath composed of mind' corresponds to the mental body and is nourished by words, images and emotions; it is dominated by the more superficial activities of our minds. The sheath consists of the thoughts and emotions that accompany us throughout our daily activities, whether it be planning tonight's dinner, negotiating the traffic or worrying about the welfare of our children.
4. The *vijnana-maya-kosha* or literally 'the sheath composed of awareness' corresponds to the psychic body and consists of deeper forces of our personality and the workings of the unconscious mind.
5. The *ananda-maya-kosha* or literally 'the sheath composed of bliss' is known as the spiritual body. It is held to be our essential nature and is said to lie beyond the states of waking, dreaming and deep sleep.

> '[Yoga] is fundamentally an energetic view of the human being in which it is impossible to separate one aspect of ourselves from the others'

Thus we can see that in yoga the human being is understood as a complex whole, with all the various sheaths influencing each other. It is fundamentally an energetic view of the human being and in this view it is impossible to separate one aspect of ourselves from the other levels. Thus physical illness may be a manifestation of disturbance at the level of our emotions or the tip of an iceberg whose roots lie in an underlying attitudinal problem. In order to allow healing, especially of persistent physical symptoms and serious illness, we may need to look beyond the physical realm. Am I feeling emotionally constipated in my life? Are there aspects of my behaviour over which I seem to have little control and which do not serve me? Do I feel animated and at peace with my friends and family? Am I able to express myself in the world freely and authentically? In the yogic world-view these different parts of our lives are seen as a whole, having intimate connections and influencing each other. Thus in order for healing to take place a holistic approach is fundamental.

In this context I was struck by how many of the individuals interviewed for this book had come to the same conclusion. Sometimes it was hinted at in their interviews and at other times it was directly stated. Anna's elegant description of how she understands the multidimensional nature of healing, so obviously imbued with her hard-won experience, affirms the wisdom of the ancients as described in yogic texts.

'I see healing as being a very multifaceted thing. I had to take into account that I've got a physical level and emotional level, a mental level a spiritual level ... It doesn't matter on what level you can work. You might be able to work on all of those levels, but each of those levels overlaps and leads into and influences the other levels. So that on whatever level you can work, whatever feels right at the time for you, you work on it knowing that it will help the other areas. There might be some times when you can work on all of those levels or there might be some times when one of those areas is so raw or so wounded that you can't touch it, so you've got to work through one of the other levels.'

I find Anna's thoughts on the process of healing particularly useful for several reasons. Firstly, she immediately acknowledges that a holistic approach that addresses the different aspects of human experience is essential. Secondly, Anna points out that each person's journey will be highly individual. And, finally, she realises that all four levels of human experience are fundamentally interrelated. She presents us with an approach to healing that allows room for our intuition but which also emphasises the need for a comprehensive appraisal of ourselves.

The gift of illness

'It is a gift, this is life saying to you, "This is the best way that we good spiritual forces know to help you learn and grow."'
ANNA RIVERS

The idea that being afflicted with a major illness could be a gift is provocative for most people. How can the loss of one's cherished livelihood or experiencing years of chronic pain be conceived in positive terms? Yet this is one of the major themes that emerges from the eight people interviewed. None of the eight describes their experience of illness as being easy, but for all of them it has been a rewarding journey. As Janelle Meisner says: 'I am much richer now in every way than I ever was before.' In this chapter I would like to explore how so many of the individuals who contributed to this book have come to the conclusion that illness can be viewed in this light.

Through successfully living with the HIV virus for more than 21 years, Peter de Reuter is well equipped to answer this question. In the Seventies, when all his friends had gurus, Peter describes feeling left out because he had never been able to find one he felt comfortable with. Then in a remarkable shift in understanding he realised that the HIV virus was his guru. With this insight Peter was able to move forward into the experience of illness and accept rather than fight his condition. As he points out, 'You can use your condition to either grow from or to become totally self-absorbed and indulgent.'

This sentiment is echoed by Shankardev Saraswati who advocates using illness '... as a springboard into higher awareness and understanding of life'. Both Shankardev and Peter speak of 'using' the illness. The word 'use' indicates a radical shift in perception. The experience of the illness, whatever its nature, then becomes grist for the mill on our journey through life. It is embraced as an important life experience – as important as any other – that has come our way and from which we can learn.

For some, however, illness as an experience is utterly indigestible. It may leave them feeling embittered and angry at God or whoever they feel is responsible for their misery. Others may simply become depressed and lose their capacity to believe that life can ever really satisfy them. Still others, as Peter suggests, entrenched in their position as a victim of illness, use their condition to manipulate their friends and family into catering for their every need. These paths, which we may wander down at some point in our struggle to get well, can fundamentally retard and sometimes prevent healing, as Peter points out.

Yet for others illness is a liberating process that makes possible a deeper level of connection to others as well as ourselves. For Rebecca Hutchinson, one of the positive aspects of being sick was having to be dependent on other people and the government. Having to receive financial assistance from the Department of Social Security was profoundly humbling for Rebecca, given that her philosophy at the time of her illness was based around being strong and independent in the world. These experiences were a catalyst for Rebecca to see how she had in the past tended to see a difference between herself and other people. As a result of this difference she would feel sympathy for other people's suffering, though sometimes would be repulsed by their pain. Ultimately, the experience of illness has enabled her to be more empathetic and more able to be with their pain and as she says, '... it's a damned fine thing to realise you're human ...'

For Anna Rivers the experience of a psychotic breakdown and its healing over a period of eight years has brought her to a deep understanding of life and the healing journey. At no point does she deny that the journey involves suffering; for Anna serious illness is a call to be a warrior. As a warrior you will be tested in many ways and this will require different qualities at different times. As she goes on to say: 'You've got to rest at times and you've got to go with the flow sometimes. You've got to understand when you've had enough, but when you can, you just fight. You don't give up.'

In this sense the experience of illness becomes a vehicle for learning about life. Inherent in this process of learning is making mistakes. Anna uses the elegant analogy of her students preparing for their first eisteddfod and the expectations they bring to their first performance. Like her students, many of us, consciously or not, will aim for a perfect performance – hoping that things will go smoothly for us in our passage through life. For Anna, our journey through life is not about a perfect performance – however we as individuals might conceive that. Rather it is an opportunity to learn, and this learning will lead us towards wholeness and peace of mind. For Anna, the ultimate kind of healing brings us to a state of complete self-acceptance and self-love.

'The journey of healing for Peter is a defining search for meaning in how to live one's life'

If one looks to the experience of Peter de Reuter over almost two decades of living with the HIV virus, one gets a strong sense of the kind of healing Anna is talking about. Peter recalls how at the time he contracted the virus he had very little self-worth and was living a destructive life using sex as a drug to blot out his emotional pain. In this context contracting HIV, as he relates, was '... the ticket that I wanted to get off this plane of reality'. Peter then relates how, by using an essentially holistic approach and addressing all four quadrants of healing, he has been able to maintain good health and to use his condition to grow from unconscious levels. The journey of healing for Peter is thus a defining search for meaning in how to live one's life: 'You need to change entirely how you think of yourself, how you live your life, how you eat, how you sleep, how you entertain. It's a call to a revolution in who you are.'

Bringing the gift into daily life

When listening to the tape recordings of the interviews, one of the most striking things is the amount of laughter I heard. Rather than being confronted with grim stories of suffering told through tense and serious faces I was met with a lightness that comes through in many of those telling their story. This capacity to see the humour in the midst of our struggles seems to be an important ingredient in how many of the individuals interviewed have worked with their illness. By seeing themselves as part of a bigger picture, they have been able to move beyond the myopic viewpoint that precluded a more humorous attitude to life. Anna Rivers brings some light to bear on this process when she talks about the process of integration that comes with healing. As she becomes more integrated she is more able to see the shades of grey in different life predicaments. The possibility of humour then becomes available to her and deters her from going down a path of self-pity or self-torture, which would diminish her ability to be with her current situation. As Anna says, 'When a person can laugh about aspects of their illness or their healing process, what a healing thing in itself that is.'

Laughter as the best medicine was an approach taken by Norman Cousins in healing himself of ankylosing spondylitis, a debilitating and painful disease that affects the spinal column. In his book *Anatomy of an Illness* he tells of how he organised screenings of Marx brothers' films from his bedside in hospital as part of his therapy.

Another theme that comes through with remarkable consistency is how the individuals are more able, since their illness, to appreciate the simple things in life. Rather than being focused on having the right car, wearing the right clothes and other material pursuits, many speak of being more able to simply enjoy being with friends or taking a walk on the beach. Sara Chesterman speaks of a restlessness that was inherent in her life prior to having her accident, a restlessness that produced a busy lifestyle in which she found herself with little time to enjoy simple things. For Peter de Reuter, sitting on a rock by his favourite little beach or enjoying the privacy of his own home are powerful ways for him to rejuvenate and to connect with, what he calls, source or God.

Many of those interviewed talk of a change in their priorities. For Sara Chesterman, it is finding your core values and then shifting your life to fulfil those values. This change in perspective is reflected in how they choose to spend their leisure time and where they decide to live, as well as the kinds of people they choose to be with. Janelle Meisner talks of coming out from her experience of chronic fatigue with a much clearer sense of what was important in her life and who her friends were. Rather than getting caught up in trying to satisfy other people's needs she was able, through her experience of illness, to develop her ability to set goals for herself and stick to them; a skill that helped her overcome her illness.

Rebecca Hutchinson also speaks of significant changes to her lifestyle as a result of getting sick. Before her illness she would hang out with people she judged to be robust, and now she is attracted to people who are more able to be with their vulnerability. Prior to her illness she went rock climbing on her weekends whereas now she draws as much pleasure from reading a good book in front of the fire at her home in the mountains.

For many of those interviewed, the experience of illness has been a powerful vehicle for 'coming into a relationship with who you really are rather than who you think you should be or who other people think you should be,' as Rebecca tells us. In the course of her illness Rebecca, like Peter de Reuter, came to see it as her teacher – a powerful guide towards a life she would otherwise have been unable to create for herself; a life she could only imagine, not actualise, prior to becoming ill.

Illness as a pathway to greater self-acceptance is a powerful theme that runs through the experience of many, if not all, of those who have contributed to this book. Shankardev Saraswati speaks of the deep insights into his own nature that have come through his experience of illness, of learning to accept himself and with this self-acceptance being able to live his life more authentically and with a greater sense of freedom. 'To live out the drama of it, the scenario, the scenes, whatever arises, and then to share whatever I've got with others.' As Shankardev has experienced serious illness first hand and successfully cured it, he is now better equipped to guide and support his patients in their own journeys through illness. In this way the experience of illness for Shankardev has brought more empathy for the plight of his patients and one suspects a far more satisfying experience of his work as a doctor.

That the experience of illness can be viewed in such positive terms, whereby it acts as a catalyst for finding meaning in one's life, is a tribute to the individuals interviewed in this book. If, like Anna, we are able to take heed from the good spiritual forces in our lives then the journey of healing through a major illness can be a powerful opportunity for learning – learning to accept ourselves, not as we would like to be, but more a warts and all acceptance that includes all the different facets of what it means to be a human being.

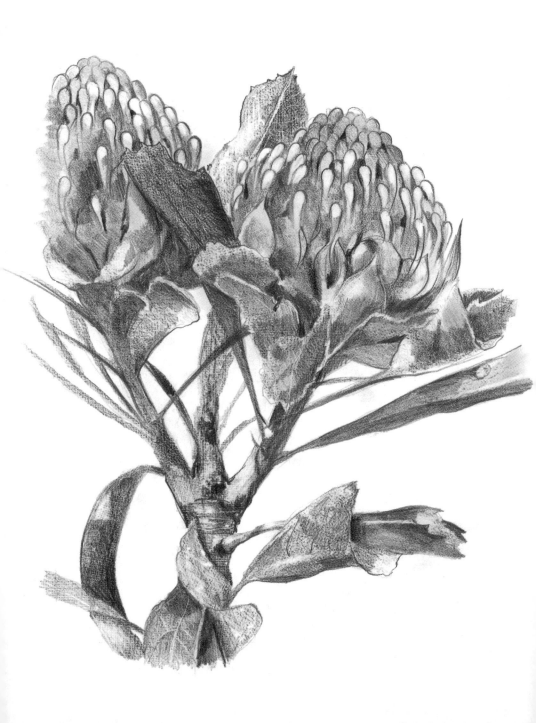

A physician's own experience

PART III

Flowers of the Australian waratah, symbolising the fruition of the healing process and flourishing growth at a time of wellness

Beyond medical school

My first encounter with the world of complementary medicine took place in a rather unexpected way during my last year in high school. My father and a few of his friends had decided to undertake a four-day whitewater canoeing trip through a wilderness area outside Sydney. The trip was not without its hazards and I was very proud, as a seventeen-year-old, to have been included in the party. The access to the river involved carrying two-man Canadian canoes down a 300-metre spur. The son of one of my father's friends had offered to assist with carrying the canoes, loaded full with watertight drums containing our provisions. Hamish, then in his late twenties, drove down with my father and me from Sydney to the site of our entry into the national park.

Hamish came from a respected rural family who owned a farm not far from where the trip was to begin. His manner was at once friendly and down to earth and during the three-hour car trip he talked freely about his work and passions in life. Despite the fact that he had been educated at one of Australia's most prestigious schools, he made his way through life as a baker of biodynamic bread. He explained how the bread was made from organically grown ingredients and instead of using yeast the bread was leavened using a honey and fruit ferment. Each morning he would bake the bread and several afternoons each week he would deliver it himself to a dozen or so health food shops in Sydney.

As well as explaining to us the health-giving benefits of food grown and prepared using biodynamic principles, Hamish also gave us a brief introduction into anthroposophy – the philosophy of Rudolph Steiner, an Austrian visionary who wrote in the 1920s about subjects as diverse as colour, medicine, agriculture and education. There was a freshness about the ideas presented to us that immediately appealed to me. My final exams at high school were still six months away and I was desperately hoping to get into medicine, even if the chances of that seemed remote at that time. What impressed me about Hamish was that he had followed his passion and was working as a baker, despite the fact that he could easily have pursued much more high-paying and high-status careers in other fields. As someone interested in having skill in the treatment of disease, it seemed entirely logical to me that to have a knowledge of both orthodox and complementary medicine could only benefit one's patients. I quietly resolved to study complementary medicine after I had finished my study of orthodox medicine, should I somehow find a place in medical school.

> '... it seemed entirely logical to me that to have a knowledge of both orthodox and complementary medicine could only benefit one's patients'

As it turned out, it would be another thirteen years before I would follow my resolve and begin my formal study of complementary medicine. In the interim I studied hard and was later accepted into the Royal College of Surgeons in Ireland – a very traditional medical school where the words 'alternative medicine' were never mentioned during my entire time of study! The clinical training, however, was excellent and I endeavoured to make the most of my six years in Dublin. The teaching hospital I was assigned to was located in the heart of the inner city and peopled with characters straight from the novels of James Joyce, so life as a medical student was never dull.

After my graduation I returned to Australia and spent two and a half years working as a hospital doctor as part of my internship and training as a resident medical officer. However, after almost nine years in the 'system' and the fatigue that comes with the long hours of hospital work I was starting to feel like a medical automaton. Having seen how dreary and boring a lot of my senior colleagues had become, and in need of some time-out, I decided to take a year off from my career in medicine. A lot of my colleagues at the time were shocked at my decision. One stopped me in the corridor of the hospital and asked me earnestly, 'Shaun, do you think you'll ever practise medicine again?' Obviously for them, taking time out from one's path through the teaching hospitals was tantamount to career suicide. Despite the occasional doubting voice, the antidote to the dehumanising influences of this environment, I had decided, was to spend a few months enjoying *la bonne vie* in the south of France. So I enrolled in a course in French language in a picturesque university town, Aix-en-Provence. Happily for me, sipping cafe-au-laits on the Cour Mirabeau, the beautiful tree-lined main street of the town, and numerous sorties into the surrounding countryside did the trick. After four months in Aix I again felt like a human being and was ready for the next stage in my adventure in medicine.

Seeing a different way

When my plane touched down in Delhi airport at around six in the morning, the captain informed us that the air temperature outside was 36 degrees Celsius and the visibility, due to dust, was down to 150 metres. This was my introduction to India in the hot season. As a result of a chance meeting with an effervescent young Australian doctor who had spent a year working with Tibetan people in Ladakh, northern India, I had arranged to spend six months working for the Tibetan government in exile at a small hospital in the foothills of the Himalayas in India. Dharamsala, located halfway up a huge spur that ascends from the plains of India to one of the first ranges of the Himalayas, has been home to His Holiness the Dalai Lama and some 9,000 Tibetan refugees since 1959.

Dharamsala is a breathtakingly beautiful place, surrounded as it is by mountains clad in rhododendron and pine forests and whose lower slopes are terraced with cornfields and dotted with the occasional villages of the local Kadhi hill tribes and brightly coloured Buddhist monasteries. It is certainly a welcome escape from the heat and dust of the Indian plains, and was a popular hill station for the British during their occupation of India. Living and working among the Tibetan refugees in Dharamsala and its surrounds gave me a wonderful entrée into their culture and Tibetan Buddhism. Many of our patients at Delek Hospital, where the doctors and nurses had been trained in Western medicine, also came under the care of the local Tibetan medicine physicians. One day, hoping to get an insight into another way of viewing health and disease, I asked a man whom I was treating for an upper respiratory tract infection what the Tibetan doctors had diagnosed. His immediate response, as relayed through the Tibetan nurse cum interpreter, was 'Too much *rlung*.'

Rlung is not an easy thing to translate into English, as I was soon to discover; the nurse broke into giggles when I asked her what this meant. Some time later I learnt that *rlung* is wind energy and an aggravation of *rlung* humour was thought to be causing this man's symptoms. In order to redress my ignorance of this approach to healing, a visit to the Tibetan Medical and Astrological Institute and its small hospital was organised.

Versed as I was in the Western scientific approach to the diagnosis of diseases and how they are caused, it took a while for me to get my head around the fact that in local Tibetan medical college students study astrology hand in hand with medicine. After ten years of approaching the field of health and disease from a modern medical perspective, to learn that the major tools in diagnosis in Tibetan medicine were feeling the pulse and looking at urine samples was challenging in itself. Looking at the ancient Tanka paintings enumerating the Tibetan system of diagnosis and treatment of diseases, I got a sense of this ancient tradition of healing and also how foreign it was to the way of thinking that I had been schooled in. For the time being my energies were more focused on dealing with the day-to-day running of the small hospital and learning about the Tibetans' unique approaches to the matter of living and dying.

One of the duties of the doctors at Delek Hospital, a 30-bed hospital run by the Tibetan government in exile, was to sleep in the hospital every fourth night and be on hand for any nocturnal emergencies. During my time there, there were five doctors on staff; three Indian-trained Tibetan doctors and two Australian doctors. When I arrived at work one morning, Peter, the other Australian doctor, related to me an unusual event that had taken place the night before.

One of our sickest patients was a Tibetan lama who was suffering from severe heart and lung failure. We had both been concerned about him because he was not responding well to treatment. Most of the time I had seen him in the wards he had been gasping for air and we did not expect him to live long. Peter had been on duty the previous night and had been writing up some medical notes from the previous day when he heard the sounds of laughter and spirited conversation in Tibetan coming from the ward where the sick lama was staying. After three-quarters of an hour three monks who were friends of the sick man left his room and returned to their monastery. Peter, on hearing the jocularity of the interchange and concerned that the monks may not have realised the seriousness of their friend's condition, asked the charge sister what had been said. In a matter-of-fact tone she replied that they had come to say goodbye to their friend and to wish him the best of luck in his next birth. Several hours later, in the early hours of the morning, the monk died, or, in Tibetan Buddhist terms, shrugged off his physical body. In an unexpected and very real way we had both been privy to a sacred tradition and its peoples that would serve to stretch our own world-view.

Both Peter and I had learnt how to meditate as medical students and were intrigued by Tibetan Buddhism and its practices. Living and working beside Tibetans gave us wonderful opportunities to see how their spiritual beliefs impacted on their lives.

Another part of our work was to visit outlying monasteries and to treat the monks, many of whom had had horrific experiences at the hands of the Chinese military in Tibet. This afforded us some intimate insights into the lives of these hardy people. At one point, concerned over how best to approach the treatment of pain in dying patients in a Buddhist community, I discussed my unease with the senior Tibetan doctor at the hospital. His immediate response was to organise for a local *geshe* or Tibetan priest to come to the hospital and discuss with the doctors how to approach these practical issues from a Buddhist perspective.

I mention all this because I can now see that the experiences I was having in Dharamsala over those months were making a powerful impression on my psyche. In combination with my own personal practice of meditation, as irregular as it was at that time, I started to open to a different way of conceptualising the treatment of disease. Initially the process was largely unconscious, but as time went on I started to relate to the human body in more energetic terms. The health of human beings seemed to be a much more complex process than I had been taught in medical school. Intuitively I knew that our mind and emotions had a significant effect on our physical health and I was convinced that meditation could profoundly influence our sense of wellbeing and resistance to disease. Although how meditation could do this was still something of a mystery to me at that time. I would need to wait a little before this piece of the jigsaw puzzle would be revealed to me.

Searching for the full story

On my return to Australia I decided it was time to experience the world of general practice and set about doing locums across the length and breadth of Sydney. It was not long before I became aware of the limitations of my training in medicine. Most of the time I felt confident in diagnosing and prescribing treatments to my patients, but every now and then a patient would come along whose set of symptoms did not fit into any of the diagnostic categories I had studied at medical school. Often I would find myself agreeing with the patient that there was definitely something wrong with their health but I could not say what it was. Concerned that I might be missing something potentially serious I would order a standard series of blood tests. Somewhat apologetically I would reassure the patient that I could find no serious cause for their symptoms and that their blood tests were all normal. We would agree to see each other in a few weeks' time to see if any of their symptoms had worsened. This whole situation was most unsatisfactory for me, and even more perplexing when a friend of mine who was a trained naturopath was easily able to diagnose some of the problems. Ultimately, I came to appreciate that there were some mild but important illnesses that had not reached the level of serious disease, which had not been properly elucidated in medical school. While my education had been sound, I had not been given the full story.

Ironically, it was during my stay in Dharamsala that I first heard of the work being done in the field of healing by an Australian man by the name of Ian Gawler. Shortly after graduating in veterinary science Ian had been diagnosed with bone cancer, which despite surgery, radiotherapy and chemotherapy had spread throughout his body. Under the guidance of a Melbourne psychiatrist, Dr Ainslie Meares, Ian had used meditation in conjunction with various complementary medicines to heal himself from what had been diagnosed as terminal cancer. His book, *You Can Conquer Cancer*, I had seen briefly in Dharamsala of all places, so I decided to visit Ian and his wife Gayle on my return to Australia. In November 1989, I joined a group of 30 cancer patients and their primary caregivers on a ten-day healing retreat. It would be my first real experience of the power of complementary medicine.

On the first morning of the retreat around fifty participants sat in a large circle at a small conference centre in a room overlooking the verdant Yarra Valley outside Melbourne. After an introduction by Ian we were all asked to tell the rest of the group why we were there. Slowly we worked our way around the group, some of the patients bearing visible scars of their battles with cancer thus far. As I listened to the heartfelt expression of stories of suffering and loss, I started to feel waves of grief move up through my chest. It seemed as if the space in the centre of the circle had become a vacuum drawing forth the emotional pain of the assembled participants.

By the time it was my turn I could barely manage to get my words out, my throat was so choked with emotion. It was clear that I had some healing of my own to do, though this had certainly not been on my agenda when I first entertained the idea of coming to see how the Gawlers worked with cancer patients. By the fourth day of the retreat the unresolved grief I had been carrying for my younger brother, who had been tragically killed in a car accident six years previously, had surfaced spontaneously. I remember spending a memorable hour by myself one morning in a grassy field reconnecting with my brother amidst some cleansing tears. There was also the clear and unequivocal realisation that for lots of 'good' reasons I had never allowed myself to properly grieve my brother's death.

Over the next ten days I was given a wonderful insight into the nature of healing. During the retreat I shared a room with a man with cancer of the oesophagus; a dairy farmer whose wife had cancer; and a father who had recently lost his teenage son to malignant melanoma, a type of skin cancer. This afforded me a unique opportunity to see into the lives of people affected by cancer in one way or another and to witness at close quarters the ups and downs of their struggles to overcome the disease. The Gawlers' approach, at that time, was based around the three pillars of a predominantly raw food diet, meditation and attitudinal healing. I also had the opportunity to meet a number of practitioners of complementary medicine who helped to support the Gawlers' programs, among them spiritual healers, meditation teachers, naturopaths and bodyworkers. All in all, despite the fact that I was in excellent physical health, it was a time of intense healing in my own life and I came away with the distinct impression that I had learnt more about healing in those ten days than I had during my six years in medical school.

On my return to Sydney, in need of a place from which to work, I set up a holistic medical centre with a group of friends who were also at the beginning of their professional lives. Our practice included another doctor, a naturopath, an acupuncturist, a psychologist and myself. It was during the next few years, in the context of general practice that I had the opportunity to meet some wonderful teachers, most of whom came to me as patients.

I remember working one balmy summer afternoon in my consulting rooms when a bearded tradesman came in to see me. Tom recounted his story of being dogged for many years by a flu-like illness, which had defied the diagnostic powers of his doctors. During this recurrent illness both his liver and spleen would enlarge causing him considerable abdominal discomfort. Finally he was referred to a specialist who recommended he undergo extensive tests in hospital. At one point during his stay in hospital, when the cause of his illness was still a mystery to his medical team, he was visited by a medical student. Rather unusually, the medical student was also studying iridology and asked if he could examine Tom's irises. After a quick look he asked if Tom was suffering from a problem with his immune system. Three weeks later, after thousands of dollars of blood tests and scans, his medical team diagnosed a rare form of immune deficiency which runs in families. Not surprisingly, my interest in the diagnostic powers of iridology was stimulated!

Even more curious were Tom's own observations of his irises after that time. In animated fashion he went on to relate to me how he would watch his irises whenever he felt that he was going to get sick. At these times a small dark spot would appear at seven o'clock in his right iris, then as he got sicker the spot would increase in size and later gradually reduce as he recovered. As Tom used to have several bouts of the illness each year, he had had ample opportunity to observe his irises in the bathroom mirror each morning and had become an avid admirer of iridology. The fact that such a simple bedside examination could be usefully employed in the diagnosis of illness was impressive and I decided to begin my own study of iridology. Several years later I went on to study iridology more formally at a college of natural therapies in Sydney and include it in the routine examination of patients who come to see me in my clinic.

Embracing the ego – psychotherapy and bodywork

I was now in my early thirties and had not been able to stay in a relationship with a woman for more than a year. On the advice of a colleague whom I had seen for an astrological consultation I decided to undertake some introductory courses in psychotherapy. It seemed that I was carrying some unconscious resistance to committing to a long-term relationship with a woman, so I thought this might be an opportunity for both learning about myself and finding more satisfaction in this area of my life. My introduction to the realm of group psychotherapy was not without its difficulties, however, as I found myself clashing with a senior psychodrama group leader. It seemed to me that there was an unhealthy dynamic at large in this group, as no-one else in the group seemed able to acknowledge my assessment of the leader's shortcomings. In the end I left the group disgruntled, and needed to debrief myself with the help of friends outside the group. As it turned out, I would have to wait some years before my perceptions of that particular community would be validated by one of its members. Despite this rather painful initial experience of group psychotherapy, I continued to pursue my interest in psychotherapy, intent as I was in getting a clearer understanding of the forces at large in my psyche. I mention this incident simply to highlight the fact that my journey into this field of learning was certainly no joy-ride and was extremely testing at times.

My interest in meditation and spiritual life was gaining momentum at this time and it made sense to me that in order to transcend the ego it was first necessary to fully embrace the ego. Psychotherapy seemed like a necessary step for me in this regard as no amount of willpower was making any difference to my love life! Having surveyed the different approaches to the art of psychotherapy on offer in Sydney at that time, I decided to undergo training in somatic or body-oriented psychotherapy. One of the underlying premises of this school of psychotherapy is that the body is a map of the unconscious – the idea that the way we hold ourselves, our posture, muscle tone and even the quality of our tissues fundamentally reflect our experiences since the time of conception. The living being is seen as a bodymind complex whereby the mind and body are dynamically interlinked and interdependent. This concept had immediate appeal for me, especially after my experiences with Tibetan medicine and through my personal experiences in meditation. It seemed wholly appropriate that many of the teachers in the course in somatic psychotherapy, while formally trained in Western psychology and psychotherapy, were also influenced by a number of Eastern spiritual traditions, including Buddhism and yoga.

One of the requirements of the training program was to have your own personal psychotherapy. One of the tenets of this kind of psychotherapy was that your effectiveness as a psychotherapist was ultimately dependent on how much you have worked with your own personal issues. As an adjunct to the work I was doing with my psychotherapist it was also suggested that I have some bodywork. In bodywork the therapist uses the power of touch to move blocked energies in the body in health-giving ways. As many of us suppress a lot of emotional energy, this energy tends to get locked into different parts of our bodies, which we experience as physical and/or emotional discomfort. My own experience, in a very real way, tended to affirm this concept.

> '... your effectiveness as a psychotherapist was dependent on how much you had worked with your own personal issues'

The bodyworker I was referred to practised a modified form of Kahuna massage, an ancient massage practice from Hawaii. He was not much older than myself and I was immediately struck by his gentle and respectful presence. Manish's approach was smooth and flowing; he barely said a word during our session, which lasted an hour and a half. In ways I still have trouble understanding, he quietly set about loosening the bands of tightness in my body, which had become my day-to-day experience of having a body and what that feels like. I particularly remember how tenderly he massaged between my toes and it was not long before the energies of my body started to dance under his nurturing touch. During the massage there was no sense of any underlying sexual agenda on his part and I felt safe enough to allow myself to let the energy move as it wanted to. This free flow of energy was accompanied by a growing sense of wellbeing and moments of bliss.

It was during my second session of bodywork with Manish that I was again reminded of the power of our emotions on our physical body. He had begun to work with my chest; placing both his hands underneath the ribs of my back he gently pulled upwards and outwards. At that moment I felt as if my lungs were sponges full of water, and as he pulled upwards it was as if he was squeezing the sponges with his hands, releasing the congealed tears held in my lungs. I could feel my diaphragm releasing as waves of grief passed through my torso. Again I was reunited with the acute sense of loss I felt for my dead younger brother but in a way that was deeply satisfying, the experience tinged as it was with the twin sisters joy and sorrow.

The fact that I might be holding some blocked energy in my chest was given further confirmation from another field of complementary medicine. One of my colleagues at the holistic medical centre practised Traditional Chinese Medicine and was skilled in the art of pulse diagnosis. Intrigued by this ancient science, I would visit John whenever I was feeling stressed or fatigued. After feeling my pulses at the beginning of the consultation John would often ask me whether I had any problems with my lungs. As someone who exercised regularly and did not smoke I would invariably reply that my lungs felt fine. He however consistently found that my pulses showed a problem with the energy in the lungs and would ask if I was conscious of feeling a lot of grief at the time of our consultations.

Ayurveda – a science of life

Up to this point I had been exposed to various approaches to maximising health and wellbeing through diet, though had never been fully convinced by any one approach in particular. From my study of iridology I had come to appreciate the importance of each individual's constitution and the bearing that this can have on one's health. It was apparent to me, even from the experience of my flatmates and close friends that no one diet suited everyone. Given my passion for meditation and the fact that yoga and Ayurveda are closely linked, I set about familiarising myself with this ancient healing tradition.

The fact that Ayurveda places great emphasis on understanding each individual's body-type and uses food as medicine also spurred my interest. With the help of some introductory books on the subject I set about modifying my diet in line with the principles of Ayurveda. What was particularly exciting to me was the fact that Ayurveda was not just a system of medicine but a complete science of life. Within this science, originally propounded by enlightened seers in India over 5,000 years ago, the role of subjective experience has always been honoured. Ayurveda is thus a meditative science, in the sense that these seers utilised the experience of their five senses and their whole bodies in their understanding of health and disease. Intuition, in this context, is seen as a God-given gift to be cultivated and used to inform one's understanding of how living creatures function. Ayurvedic understanding of the treatment of disease is also informed by the empirical experience of Ayurvedic practitioners over several millenia.

It was not long before I had my own experience of the benefits of the Ayurvedic approach to diet. Over the years I had come to recognise how certain foods did not agree with me and had stopped having chilli, coffee and rich foods, so it was affirming to find that the diet appropriate for my Ayurvedic constitution suggested that such foods should be avoided as they could lead to health imbalances for my particular body-type.

Around this time I started to get the sense that here was a system of medicine and healing that encompassed the full range of human experience. Yet the opportunities for further study seemed limited. Keen to have an authentic experience of Ayurveda I wrote off to the Indian Embassy in Canberra and was given a list of Ayurvedic colleges in India. Out of the fifteen colleges I applied to only one had an English medium course. Excited at the prospect of continuing my study in this ancient healing tradition, I headed off to the small town of Jamnagar in Gujarat, the state where Mahatma Gandhi was born.

Gujarat Ayurved University was established in the 1950s at a time when India's leaders were keen to promote India's indigenous arts and sciences. It is India's only university exclusively devoted to Ayurveda and has both undergraduate and postgraduate courses. Jamnagar is a quiet and dusty town, well off the beaten track, which draws Ayurvedic physicians from all over India to its highly regarded MD and PhD courses. Despite the old-fashioned teaching styles, Jamnagar proved to be an excellent place to immerse myself in Ayurveda. All my fellow students in the intensive course for foreign medical professionals were from Sri Lanka and they generously shared their knowledge of Ayurveda, which is also strong in Sri Lanka.

I soon realised that I was the only Westerner living in Jamnagar and within weeks had become something of a celebrity in the town. Total strangers called out to me in the streets in friendly fashion, many clearly impressed that here was a Westerner studying India's own system of medicine. Meals at the Postgraduate Ayurvedic Boys Hostel were always a treat with four different messes to choose from. As most Ayurvedic physicians are very particular eaters, the dining hall had both North and South Indian messes as well as the local Gujarati and Maharashtran messes. Each mess had a cook whose job it was to produce fresh and well-prepared food for her fold. It was at mealtimes that I started to realise the extent to which Ayurveda is sown into the fabric of many of the cultural practices of India and how it informs the Indian approach to the preparation and selection of food. The idea that food and kitchen herbs could be used medicinally was starting to gain substance in my own mind.

During my stay in Jamnagar I came into contact with Ayurvedic physicians from all over India, many of whom came from families who had been practising Ayurveda for centuries. Dr Ganapathi Bhat, from the state of Karnataka in South India, was one such Ayurvedic physician. His family has a documented Ayurvedic medical tradition, which has been passed down from generation to generation for over 400 years. The fact that Ayurvedic knowledge had been kept alive, particularly in the South, as part of an oral tradition impressed me and a few years later I undertook an Ayurvedic study tour of South India with Ganapathi and one of his colleagues. As I learnt more about Ayurveda I realised that to study it in isolation would be to do it a disservice. Just as I had studied anatomy, physiology and biochemistry together in medical school, I now understood the necessity of studying Ayurveda, yoga and Vedic astrology, as sister sciences. I had observed this at the Tibetan Medical and Astrological Institute in Dharamsala some six years previously.

Yoga and Vedic astrology

I had been introduced to yoga several years previously and had come to appreciate yoga postures as wonderful tools in relieving accumulated stress from the body. At first my yoga practice had been periodic but under the guidance of one of my colleagues in Australia, who was a yoga teacher as well as a medical practitioner, I started to see how it could be harnessed in the treatment of disease. While in Jamnagar I decided to commit to a daily practice of yoga postures and it was not long before I came to appreciate the subtle effects of even ten minutes of yoga exercises on one's physiology and energy levels. Keen to expand my knowledge of this companion to Ayurveda, several years later I again returned to India to study at the Bihar School of Yoga in Mongier. In this tradition considerable emphasis is given to the study and practice of all different aspects of yoga. As well as yoga postures, breathing exercises and meditation, we were introduced to the yoga of selfless service, also known as karma yoga. The Bihar School of Yoga is well known in India for the excellent quality of its books and research in the application of yoga in the treatment of common medical conditions, including diabetes, high blood pressure and asthma.

While living in Sydney, strange as it may seem, I had the opportunity of furthering my understanding of Ayurveda, through an introductory study of Vedic astrology or *Jyotish*. In the mid-Nineties, Hart de Foux was invited by my friend and colleague, Dr Shankardev Saraswati, to come and teach Vedic astrology in Sydney. Hart is Canadian by birth and had a fifteen-year apprenticeship with a master of Vedic astrology in India. He now travels the world for six months of the year doing consultations and teaching *Jyotish*. My understanding of yoga and Vedic astrology have gone a long way to providing an appropriate context for my practice of Ayurveda.

I have also spent time studying various forms of Ayurvedic massage and its deep cleansing techniques, called *Panchakarma*, as these are fundamental therapeutic arms of Ayurveda.

While in Jamnagar, one of my teachers, Professor Kulwant Singh, advised me that patient education would be one of my first priorities in getting Ayurveda established in Australia. Accordingly, on my return to Sydney, Shankardev and I started running ten-week courses in Ayurveda as a science of self-healing. Each Wednesday night around twenty people crowded into our living room, among them doctors, massage therapists, naturopaths, yoga teachers and cancer patients. Our courses became well known in Sydney, Ayurveda being relatively unknown at that time in the general population, and helped to build up our unusual medical practices.

Putting it all into practice

During the next five years I started to integrate into my clinical practice what I had learnt in India. I was fortunate to have supervision with two gifted somatic psychotherapists, which was absolutely invaluable in deepening my understanding of the human bodymind in health and disease. It also proved to be an important and necessary forum for learning how to bring Ayurvedic and yogic approaches to healing into a contemporary Western setting. The psychology of the Indian and Western mind have some important differences.

My medical practice in Sydney reflects the various healing traditions I have been exposed to. Consultations last for around an hour and, while I draw considerably from my knowledge of Western medicine, most of the treatments I offer are informed by Ayurveda and yoga. I will often find myself teaching patients gentle yoga stretches or meditation practices to help relax their bodies deeply, thereby allowing their immune systems to work optimally. It is my experience that very few people living in the city know how to relax deeply, so I make a relaxation tape with patients as part of the consultation, as an aid to encourage them to make time for rest and rejuvenation each day. A consultation will also include an assessment of their unique Ayurvedic body-type and proceed to a detailed examination of their daily food intake, routines and lifestyle. Ensuring that the patient leaves with an awareness of how to improve their own nourishment is absolutely vital to the process of healing and as such I will often prescribe kitchen herbs along with a diet appropriate for their body-type. To facilitate this process I run Ayurvedic cooking classes with a friend of mine, Tim Mitchell, a gifted Ayurvedic chef. During the seminars we luxuriate in wonderful smelling herbs and spices and the days are always a wonderful celebration of food and how to nourish oneself.

Many of the patients who come to see me are suffering from various kinds of chronic diseases and have had little success with conventional medicine. Simply put, I teach them how to maximise their health through changing their diet, lifestyle and awareness of themselves. Sometimes counselling is required to address underlying emotional issues and attitudes that are preventing healing from taking place. I will refer patients for psychotherapy if I feel there is a need for a deeper level of attitudinal healing; this process naturally requires a lot more commitment from the patient.

At the holistic medical centre where I worked from 1994 until 2001 there were four doctors as well as a dozen or so other practitioners of complementary medicine, including a naturopath, a medical herbalist, a practitioner of Traditional Chinese Medicine, an Ayurvedic physician, bodyworkers and psychotherapists of different kinds. It is not uncommon for one patient to be seeing several practitioners at our centre, which helps to ensure optimal rates of recovery from illness. Given the fact that many of the practitioners are friends, newcomers to the centre are often impressed by the inherent warmth that tends to emanate from the reception area, which is a great place for patients, receptionists and practitioners to chat. The invisible wall that so often separates doctors from their patients is not to be found here!

As reflected in this book, the patients who come for treatment at my clinic come with a broad spectrum of illnesses. Many are suffering from chronic diseases; some have exhausted the treatment options that Western medicine has to offer, while others come desirous of greater wellbeing and want to know how best to maintain their health. It is in the domain of preventive medicine that Ayurveda and yoga have much to offer. Indeed, of the eight branches of Ayurveda, two deal solely with rejuvenation of the bodymind and how to make men and women more fertile.

My job is to help people access the divine healer that exists within all of us. In practical terms I help people to expand their thinking about what is possible with their health and introduce them to simple ways in which they can maximise their own healing. Often this will involve challenging existing belief systems that are limiting their recovery and also teaching them practical skills to enhance their health. Those patients who are prepared to make changes to the way they are living their lives tend to do best. Indeed, some of the patients I have worked with who have been able to achieve profound healing were the inspiration behind putting together this book.

Physician heal thyself

For the first 35 years of my life I led what my iridology teacher described as a 'charmed' existence in terms of physical health. As such, I was not well equipped emotionally for my first encounter with ill health. It took the form of a night of intense right-sided abdominal pain, an unremitting pain I could not ignore which heralded the beginning of a difficult, though ultimately rewarding, journey of healing.

The timing of my abdominal pain is significant. It occurred a week after my return from a holiday in Sumatra with my girlfriend at that time. During our trip I had experienced a couple of days of abdominal upset and on my return to Sydney had had an episode of blood in my stool. This had responded, or so I thought, to some Ayurvedic herbs specific for dysentery. While on holiday my girlfriend and I had decided to live together and the onset of my abdominal pain coincided with the night she moved into my house.

The severity of the abdominal pain that night took me by surprise, though on reflection my bowel had not been happy for some time. For years I had been sensitive to hot spices and anything more than a glass of wine would produce some discomfort in my right side under the rib cage. During a trip to India four years previously I had overdosed on chilli and this had served to weaken my digestion. After this trip I noticed that I would experience abdominal discomfort after meals and when feeling emotionally stressed. The type of emotional stress seemed to be particularly related to times of intense frustration or when feeling attacked by people whom I encountered in life.

Six weeks after the onset of this abdominal pain, three amoebic ulcers of my large bowel were formally diagnosed during a colonoscopic examination by my gut specialist. I was most grateful for this diagnosis, given the worry I had been experiencing when not knowing what was going on. My training in medicine did nothing to allay my fear about my diagnosis. The pervasive nature of this fear was something I could not possibly have appreciated prior to my own experience of having an undiagnosed and painful illness.

In many ways my life at the time of this episode of abdominal pain was working well, or so I thought. I lived close to the ocean, where I swam each day, and was in the midst of an exciting new romance. I had a satisfying career as a complementary medical practitioner, a great circle of friends and a rich and rewarding spiritual life inspired by nature and teachings from India. Getting sick with ulceration of my large bowel just did not make sense. I kept thinking that I was doing all the 'right' things. I had a well-balanced diet informed by the approach of Ayurveda, I practised yoga exercises each morning for half an hour, I had trained in psychotherapy and had spent three years having my own weekly therapy. Why should I get sick? When I looked around at some of my friends who drank and smoked and exercised once a month, I really struggled to understand why I should get an inflamed bowel and three ulcers. It didn't seem fair!

'The pervasive nature of this fear was something I could not possibly have appreciated prior to ... having an undiagnosed and painful illness'

Anger and confusion

For a long while after the diagnosis I was in a kind of psychic shock. Something about the whole situation did not compute and challenged a lot of beliefs I had about why people get sick. I was angry that, despite making considerable efforts to maintain good health and wellbeing in a number of different areas of my life, I had been struck down. I felt cheated and was at a loss as to how to proceed in order to best facilitate my own healing. A couple of weeks prior to having the colonoscopic examination I had consulted a naturopathic colleague who felt, while acknowledging the physical disruption to my tissues, that the source of the pain in my side was emotional. Somehow I believed that three years of body-oriented psychotherapy should have been enough to deal with disharmony between my mind and my body. It was now apparent that there was a lot more for me to learn in order for healing to take place.

At the same time that all these thoughts and feelings were circulating in my being, there were plenty of practical issues to be faced. The pain in my abdomen was made worse by sitting in a chair for more than half an hour and my medical practice, based as it was around hour-long consultations, could not be sustained. I was also forced to resign from my position as a university associate lecturer because sitting for three hours in a tutorial group had become out of the question. Fortunately, at my father's suggestion several years earlier I had taken out income disability insurance, which enabled me to cover my living expenses and the cost of visits to different health care practitioners.

What I did come to appreciate was how much of my sense of myself in the world was tied up in what I did for a living, in a way that would have been impossible for me to acknowledge prior to getting sick. I noticed within myself a concern about no longer being productive. I could no longer relate to myself in my usual way, as being a useful member of society. Somehow, with the loss of my livelihood, in my own eyes I had become driftwood. This ongoing sense of feeling less than others became a dominant subtext in my life that I would find difficult to let go of.

During my occasional visits to the holistic medical centre where I had worked previously it was difficult for me not to feel like some kind of fraud, or at best a failure. As someone who had been teaching Ayurveda as a science of self-healing to hundreds of students, falling sick seemed to tear a big hole in my credibility as a teacher. This blow to my self-esteem was exacerbated by the offhand comment of a colleague who, on hearing of my plight asked, 'Can't you use Ayurveda to fix yourself?' At the time I could only hear her comment as: 'What's the matter with you? Why can't you heal yourself?' In the state I was in at the time, it was easy for me to feel shamed and for this colleague's comment to send me into a downward spiral of anguish.

Needless to say, the emotional turmoil I was experiencing at this time was putting a considerable strain on my fledgling relationship with my girlfriend. Prior to this relationship I had always kept my girlfriends at arm's length and had never co-habitated. The experience of living together seemed to be inordinately difficult for both of us. When I looked around it seemed that a lot of my friends enjoyed the experience of living together, particularly in the first year. What was the matter with me? A gnawing sense of shame and failure at my inability to do what other people seemed to be able to manage eroded my confidence further. Surely the work I had done on myself in the previous six years of study in communication skills and psychotherapy would have equipped me for this? My confusion rattled me to the core, and the clear and simple answers that I yearned for were not forthcoming. A month after the diagnosis of amoebic ulceration of my large bowel, in the midst of this turmoil, I decided to return to psychotherapy in search of some answers. (I speak of my experiences in psychotherapy a little later in this chapter.)

Looking for answers

The specialist I had been attending was confident that the ulcers in my bowel would respond quickly to antibiotic therapy. However, I was not so sure. As I mentioned earlier, my bowel had been out of balance for a long time. Although it seemed likely that I had picked up the amoeba while travelling through Indonesia, I was also aware that I had been prone to attacks of discomfort in the gut for several years. My condition had a long history and my understanding from studying Ayurveda and Traditional Chinese Medicine was that conditions of imbalance that have been present for a long time tend to take a long time to heal. This idea seemed to make perfect sense to me and correlates with how I understand the processes of nature. However, a part of me certainly wanted to believe the specialist. As it transpired, two courses of antibiotics over a period of a month, both highly specific for amoebic disorders, resulted in only a 50 percent improvement in my abdominal pain, the most sensitive indicator of how my bowel was faring. I realised that a more comprehensive approach to the treatment of my condition was required.

From my training in holistic healing I realised that I would need to consider all four quadrants of healing – the physical, emotional, mental and spiritual – in order to get well. The physical aspect of my health was in reasonable shape as I had kept up my 30 minutes of yoga practice each morning and swam in the ocean most days. For many years I had cooked for myself using plenty of fresh vegetables, whole grains and fruit. However, in order to give my bowel the best chance of healing I now consulted a professor of Traditional Chinese Medicine skilled in the use of Chinese herbs. The professor was a delightful man in his seventies who had immigrated to Australia a few years previously and would often ply me with food and stories of archeological digs he had been involved in in China. When I arrived at his practice one day with my dog, Jaffa, he was quick to tell me that roasted dog was one of his favourite dishes! For three months I dutifully cooked up his dried herbs in a clay pot and drank the decoction twice daily. However, despite his assurances that my condition could be cured, and to my disappointment, there was only very slight improvement over this time.

To address the emotional and mental levels of my condition I returned to psychotherapy, this time with an older female psychotherapist. After our first meeting, I felt sure she would trigger any residual issues I might have with my mother, and I was not mistaken! Most of my previous experience of psychotherapy had been with a man and though I had very little idea of what would come up in our sessions, it seemed likely that working with this woman would be a productive area of endeavour. However, rather than getting some scintillating insights into how my way of being in the world was contributing to my illness, I was soon to encounter 'real' difficulties in our work together. My armchair ride into the world of psychotherapy had ended! For one thing she did not share my understanding of the bodymind in health and disease and when she persisted in holding on to her view of the world, I was quick to self-righteously dismiss the validity of her position!

Our sessions became rather intense at times, especially after she suggested we meet twice a week in order to provoke my resistance to the therapy. She accurately pointed out that I had controlled my relationship with my mother by putting geographical distance between her and myself. When things got too hot I would simply move away – a useful strategy when you are an adolescent male but not always so useful as a man in his thirties intent on nurturing a long-term relationship! Through the work with the psychotherapist I came to see how I had been trying to live up to some kind of ideal in my relationship with my girlfriend. I realised how I had been putting myself under enormous strain trying to fulfil the requirements of how a 'good' relationship should look, in my own mind.

For a year and a half I laboured with this work and along the way gained some important, if hard-won, insights into areas of my life where how I was thinking and acting really did not serve me. I identified areas where a lot of my responses, though quite unconscious, would leave me feeling hard done by and result in my feeling unnecessary anguish. At the end of this time my abdominal pain was no longer constant but was still making it difficult for me to sit in a chair for longer than a couple of hours. Concerned about the lack of progress with my physical health, I asked the psychotherapist how much longer it would take before the issues we had touched on would be resolved. She said that, although further work would be helpful, she felt it could take several years without there being any breakthroughs in my physical health. With my bank balance shrinking and convinced that there must be a more effective way of healing these levels of my being, I decided to stop therapy.

> 'I had been putting myself under enormous strain trying to fulfil the requirements of how a "good" relationship should look'

I experienced constant pain in my abdomen, at differing levels of intensity, over a period of six months, and this had a marked effect on my mood. Socialising with friends and family became fraught with difficulty, as my abdominal pain would always become worse after meals. The only way to relieve it I had found was to go for a twenty-minute walk. Negotiating this, especially at a dinner party with people you did not know well, was for me at that time an arduous process. As well as this there were certain foods that I did not tolerate well and checking with the cook of the house about the food they were preparing became somewhat tiresome. Having to explain my specific dietary requirements and making sure that they both understood what I had said and knew what was contained in the food could sometimes be a lengthy process. It could also feel imposing from my perspective. As being sick was a reminder that I had failed in some way, public disclosures of my illness were a potential source of embarrassment. In this context I started to dread the idea of dinner parties and social engagements that would mean a lot of sitting down, something I had never previously experienced, being a naturally gregarious person at heart.

Finding help in unexpected places

In my struggle to return to what I considered good health, the first step of which was to rid my body of the nagging pain and discomfort in my side, I received an enormous amount of help along the way, often from unexpected quarters. The first of these hope-giving encounters happened a week or so before the colonoscopic examination by the gastroenterologist. I was visiting a friend of mine who was living in a small coastal town a few hours north of Sydney. David had gone through medical school with me and was working as a locum general practitioner. One of his patients, a young mother, had mentioned that she was a spiritual healer and David had told her of my interest in complementary medicine. At the time of my visit I was experiencing a lot of anxiety about the forthcoming colonoscopic examination and was fearful that the symptoms of abdominal pain and weight loss of 5 kilograms might be due to bowel cancer. When I look back now it all seems so unlikely, but at the time I was engulfed with the uncertainty of my situation. Following an intuition I decided to give this woman a call and, heartened by her warm and friendly reception on the phone, decided to see her for a session. My medical condition allowed me a licence to go places I would normally not go, for lots of 'good' reasons.

I sat with her in her living room and poured out the details of my story. She exuded a non-judgemental presence and I felt safe to tell her about my deep and seemingly irrational fears. She listened patiently throughout, and this was healing in itself. Later she communed with my spirit guides and then asked me to lie down on the carpet while she waved her arms above my body and went into what seemed to be some kind of trance-like state. During this time a lot of information and suggestions came to her about my medical condition and life situation, a lot of which it is difficult for me to remember now. However, she was able to see a blue energy coursing through my bowel, which was unobstructed, and she seemed confident that there was no cancer in my system. Strange as it may seem, I had a strong sense that what she was describing about my body was accurate, certainly the effect of the session was to considerably allay my anxiety about having cancer in my bowel. I left her house feeling strangely blessed and with a strong sense of the untold mysteries of life. When she refused to take any money for the two hours of her time I had taken up, I agreed to send her some Ayurvedic cooking recipes to help her with her family's diet. The other memorable part of the experience was when her seven-year-old son returned home from school in the middle of our session, when I was lying on the living room floor, and she calmly asked him to make himself some afternoon tea. Her son, for that matter, seemed quite unfazed by the proceedings – no doubt used to the ways of his mother!

Several months after receiving the diagnosis of illness and still struggling to comprehend why I had got sick, I had a chance encounter with a peripatetic Aboriginal healer. Gerry had recently returned from the United States and originally hailed from the area of the North Coast of New South Wales, home to the Bundjalung people. Ironically, my session with him took place in a small room on the fourth floor of a beauty school in the heart of downtown Sydney. The healers in his people's tradition had always worked with precious stones and Gerry used a lot of gemstones and crystals during his sessions. He quietly asked me to lie on a massage table and then went about cleansing my aura using a crystal rod and through some sixth sense of his identified a large hole in my etheric field and even an unneeded psychic entity that was with me. Although I could not relate to his experience of my disturbed state, Gerry radiated a deep calm, which I naturally trusted. Following this feeling, rather than getting caught up in an intellectual analysis of what he was doing, I relaxed into the unfolding experience. Using a crystal rod, Gerry said that he repaired the gaping hole in my aura and at the end of the session asked me to drink a gem elixir. The elixir was made by placing an appropriate gem stone in a glass of water and allowing it to sit in direct sunlight for half an hour.

During our session the ever-present pain in my abdomen dissolved away completely, for which I was profoundly grateful. The relief from the onslaught of pain was itself a lovely gift, but what was even more potent for me was the hope that came with the cessation of the pain. Somewhere along the track I had begun to wonder whether I would ever be able to live a pain-free existence. The fact that this man was able to remove my pain gave me an enormous amount of encouragement at the time. The last thing Gerry asked me to do was to stand up and hold out my arms in a curved manner in front of me; I naturally complied wondering what form our healing ritual would take next. He then gave me a warm and gentle hug, not what I was expecting at all but delightful to receive at a time when I was feeling unloveable and undernourished.

My session with Gerry was now over, or so I thought, however plucking up some courage I asked him one last question: 'But Gerry, why did I have to get sick?' He looked at me calmly and gently replied, 'In order to be able to help the people that come to see you, you need to have experienced sickness yourself.' Gerry's simple words, delivered with the compassion that I sensed came from great personal suffering, had a deep impact on me. Catching the crowded city bus home that afternoon, I was awash with an enormous sense of relief and the beginnings of a new understanding. Somehow, through this man's presence and words, I realised that getting sick was not my fault. A huge burden was lifted from my shoulders and I could embrace more deeply the possibility that becoming ill could be an important rite of passage in my journey into healing.

The healing that took place as a result of my last-minute question to Gerry had a serendipitous quality. I had sought Gerry's services wanting help with the chronic pain in my gut; however, what I had come away with was relief from the self-imposed burden of responsibility for my condition that I had been carrying since getting ill. During the course of my healing the role of serendipity became apparent on several occasions and at those times I would feel humbled by a wonderful sense of grace descending.

Another unexpected quarter from which I received a lot of help was in the form of a delightful practitioner of Traditional Chinese Medicine who practises in the heart of Chinatown in Sydney. Xue Min had immigrated to Australia four years previously and set up a practice with her sister who is a beauty therapist. I had spent the morning seeing another Chinese herbalist, whose shop is next door, and had noticed a small sign in Xue Min's shopfront window advertising Chinese massage in the treatment of colitis. Intrigued, I walked in and soon had a preliminary consultation with Xue Min. The style of massage she practises is very gentle and aims to improve the functioning of the internal organs, such as the liver and spleen, thereby improving digestive power and immune system functioning. The cost of the massage was relatively cheap and Xue Min delivered the massage, done through clothes on my abdomen, with a rocking motion that was very soothing. Best of all I would nearly always leave there with no pain in my belly, which always instilled confidence that a cure for my condition and a pain-free life was possible. Xue Min was a naturally caring person and always treated me with the utmost respect and gentleness, so it was always a pleasure to be in her company. I have always enjoyed the cross-cultural aspect of treatments in Chinatown, and Xue from time to time would tell me snippets of her life in Communist China, prior to emigrating, and a few details of the esoteric healing tradition that she was carrying on.

> 'I could embrace more deeply the possibility that becoming ill could be an important rite of passage in my journey into healing'

Looking inside

The eighteen months during which I had weekly psychotherapy marked a time of considerable introspection for me. Given the difficulties of socialising, which I described earlier, I found that I had become somewhat isolated and could see that this was not serving me well. Although I had a strong daily personal spiritual practice centred around the philosophy of Vedanta – in which one is involved in the inquiry, 'Who am I? Who is the thinker of these thoughts?' – I was aware that I would benefit from more spiritual community in my life. By this I mean having regular contact with like-minded people who are also committed to a spiritual path that seeks to uncover the divine in everyday life. With this in mind I started to attend a weekly meeting in some friends' home with an Australian teacher of Sanskrit and Vedanta. During these classes Michael took a group of twenty or so people through readings of ancient Hindu texts such as the Upanishads and the Bhagavad-Gita. The Friday evenings brought together a delightful mix of people of all ages and the friendly chats over hot cups of chai (sweet and spicy Indian milk tea) at the end of the night were always food for the heart. I look back on the year or so that I attended these meetings warmly and can see how important they were in helping me to regain my confidence socially and in supporting my own spiritual practice.

It is my good fortune to be the part-owner of 36 hectares of bushland on the other side of the Blue Mountains, about three hours' drive west of Sydney. The land is situated on top of a small mountain and looks out over kilometres of low, undulating hills, for the most part covered with virgin forest. It is largely uncleared and home to an array of wombats, kangaroos, wallabies and lyrebirds, to name only a few. Happily, my illness allowed me to spend a little more time in the bush, and I developed the practice of lying down under gum trees and looking up through the uppermost leaves at the sky. At one level I was practising doing nothing – not walking, not reading, not meditating, not thinking actively about anything – at another level I was just hanging out under a tree in the bush, nothing more. Still, this was enormously freeing and it allowed a passive level of contemplation from which I would emerge feeling refreshed. These moments, though infrequent, were very restorative to my spirit, especially when the tyranny of abdominal pain was starting to get to me. In tandem with a daily practice of prayer and self-inquiry, the bush was and continues to be a powerful medicine for me.

I had spent a couple of weeks up at our land and was returning to Sydney, around a year and a half after the diagnosis of my illness, when I had one of the turning points in my recovery. As I drove down through the Blue Mountains I casually grabbed an audiotape on healing from the glove box of my car and put it on. The tape had been given to me by an acquaintance who works in palliative care and featured a discussion between Ram Das and Stephen Levine. It was recorded in an AIDS ward in San Francisco in 1984, and involves an inquiry between two spiritual teachers and the patients in the ward into what they called 'the heart of healing'. Ram Das and Stephen Levine had been involved in work with the dying and the bereaved for many years in the United States and were sharing from their experience and the experience of people they had worked with. At one point Ram Das, an ex-professor of psychology from Harvard University whose life had been profoundly changed after meeting his Indian guru Neem Karoli Baba, shared his own struggle to accept his humanity. In particular he spoke of his need to be seen to be 'together' and 'in control', his need not to be vulnerable and the little corners of himself normally hidden from view because of shame. He shared how he had spent an enormous amount of time running around trying to be superhuman and had learnt that what he needed to do was to embrace all of his humanity in order to be fully human.

His words struck a profound chord in my heart as I realised the extent to which I had been doing the same thing in my own life. The timing of my listening to the tape was ideal as I was particularly open and receptive after my time of solitude. Driving down the mountain I received a powerful insight into how my approach to life up to that point in time had been denying important aspects of myself – the part of me that desperately does not want to feel needy or dependent, the part of me that is loathe to admit feeling vulnerable or out of control. That night I got a clear view of that shadowy part of myself normally hidden from view. Intellectually, I had known for many years that I needed to own my ego before trying to transcend it; now I was getting a more profound experience of what that actually means. The experience of my illness had again afforded me the opportunity of a deeper level of healing than I could have ever imagined. Again I was confronted with the awe and mystery of life and continued on my way down the mountain road with tears in my eyes and a heart full of gratitude.

Taking stock

The stillness of my time in the bush helped me to digest the experiences I had had since getting ill eighteen months previously. Taking stock of my situation I felt that I was now 80 percent recovered. I was still experiencing abdominal discomfort and was a few kilos underweight. I had resumed my work at the university, was enjoying teaching at a college of natural therapies and was being paid to develop a three-year course in Ayurvedic healing. Sadly, my girlfriend had decided to end our relationship several months before, the strain of my illness contributing to the difficulties of being together. I felt hurt and rejected and at the same time could see that in many ways we weren't very compatible for a long-term relationship. It had been a challenging experience for both of us and I also felt a sense of relief that my life had become simpler again.

It was apparent that in terms of the symptoms of my illness my progress had plateaued and that, despite having worked comprehensively at a number of different levels in my healing, further improvement was not forthcoming. Something else was required; something that addressed some deeply held attitudes in my being that were limiting my full recovery. At this point I did not know what form this kind of healing might take but stayed open to the possibility that this level of healing could be addressed, perhaps through a healing process that can come in groups – such as a men's group or some kind of twelve-step process. Happily, a few months later, while interviewing one of the contributors to this book, I was given another key piece in the jigsaw puzzle.

I had asked Nicki Youdale, whose Herculean struggle with life-threatening congenital heart disease is the subject of Nicki's story, about what had helped her most in her healing. She had mentioned a particular international personal development and training corporation, and how doing their three-day intensive course and its follow-on seminar series over three months had helped her to shift some profoundly limiting attitudes that were retarding her ability to have better health. Given my respect for Nicki as a human being, her comments immediately sparked my interest. However, it was not until I had a conversation with her sister Romaine, as a part of my research for the book, that I glimpsed the possibility that doing such a seminar could be of benefit to me. During my conversation with Romaine she spoke freely about how she had also got a lot out of doing the personal development course. She mentioned some of the principal ideas presented in the seminar and I could see immediately how they were relevant to me, particularly in my relationship with my mother.

Our relationship had become strained since the death of my father eight years previously, and despite our best efforts neither of us had been able to restore our previous closeness. At that time I was convinced that a more satisfying relationship would never be possible because, in my own mind, she had become an undermining and controlling figure in my life, around whom I would always find it difficult to feel safe. The situation seemed intractable, and while we did share some moments of connection and respect, they tended to be infrequent.

I also needed to get over some misgivings I had about the nature of the personal development course, as a brief encounter with it ten years previously had not been a positive one. After attending an introductory evening at the request of some friends I had left with the feeling that I didn't need this seminar in order to live my life successfully and, although I wouldn't have acknowledged it at the time, fearful of having to share my innermost thoughts and feelings in such a public way. This fear was still present when I decided to sign up for the seminar but I knew that the confrontation inherent in its approach was what I now needed. At some point in my development I had decided that I was 'special' or in some way above all the courses that some of my contemporaries were flocking to. Taking on this personal development course directly challenged that belief system; and although feeling uncomfortable with the prospect of doing it – 'What would all my spiritual friends think?!' – another part of me was determined to see what it had to offer and to make the most of it as an opportunity for learning. I was not to be disappointed.

Laying the groundwork for healing

The two hundred or so seminar participants were mostly seated when I walked in through the door at the front of the room carrying a lightweight futon on my shoulder. It seemed like all eyes were focused on me at that moment – 'What's he doing with a futon on his shoulder? What's the matter with him?' – my imagination was running overtime. Knowing that sitting on a chair for up to twelve hours a day for the three days of the seminar would be beyond me, I had negotiated with the management to be able to lie on my futon if the discomfort in my abdomen became too great. In this moment I would have to expose my disability before all and sundry and publicly acknowledge my vulnerability and weakness. Certainly this is how it felt as I entered the seminar hall and quickly found an out-of-the way position for my futon at the back of the room. In fact, most people hardly seemed to notice my presence after the first few hours, obviously there were many more important things at stake for them. The few comments I did get were from people rather envious of my ability to stretch when I felt like it. The healing of my shame had already started.

In this personal development course an experienced and well-trained facilitator presents a number of principles, around which the seminar is based, to the assembled participants. The participants are asked to focus on a specific area of their lives that is causing them concern and to see if the distinctions presented have relevance for them personally. The process can set up a powerful means of reflection into who you are being in your life and participants are asked to share any personal insights that come up for them during the seminar. Invariably the sharing of individual participants enlivens this process of self-reflection and in my experience sooner or later someone's story will resonate with your own. What was remarkable about this educational approach was its capacity to take people out of their habitual ways of relating to each other and themselves. In my case, on the second day of the seminar I was lying on my back looking up at the ceiling when I saw how my innate self-righteousness was destroying my relationship with my mother. Being such a fundamental relationship in life, I could also see how this way of being had placed a huge strain on all my intimate relationships. Although I did not get up to share during the three days of the seminar, I knew that I had been given a key to unlock the cell that I had placed myself in. The seminar series also provided practical ways to obviate the anguish and shame that had become all too frequent companions.

When the light of realisation dawned, it was abundantly clear to me that I owed several people in my life an apology. Most of all my mother who had been the recipient of a lot of judgement from me in previous years and who had been untiringly generous in her treatment of me. I visited her the morning after the seminar at her home and shared my insights from the previous few days and apologised to her for being such a self-righteous and judgemental son. That day we were able to connect in a very real way as we had not been able to for many years, and I had the sense that it was the most creative and loving conversation I could remember having with my mother. Certainly it heralded the beginning of a new relationship between us, which we have been able to maintain ever since.

Ultimately the personal development course helped me address in a profound way some unconscious attitudes that were blocking my development as a human being and which had not been touched during several years of psychotherapy. It provides a wonderful forum for the exchange of people's stories; people from all walks of life and of different ages. The inspiration that flows from these stories and the willingness of the participants to address old and deeply felt wounds is extraordinary.

The work I did with this organisation over the next three months provided the groundwork for healing of the attitudes I felt were impeding my full recovery. As I became more able to accept my own faults and flaws I started to be more able to accept those in other people, thereby making it possible for me to be with people in a more relaxed way – a way which importantly did not leave me feeling slighted, or at times wounded, by other people's comments or behaviour. In a way that is difficult to admit, I came to realise from doing the seminar that life had become painful for me. So it was not surprising that I had ended up with chronic physical pain!

A new way of being

After doing this seminar and its follow-up evenings my bowel condition improved gradually over the next couple of years. During this time, keen to work at the bodily level in conjunction with the mental work I was doing, I had regular bodywork with a practitioner of Ortho Bionomy. Ortho Bionomy is an approach to healing that seeks to assist the body in finding its natural alignment. By supporting the body in coming into balance, individuals are able to learn a new and innately healthy way of living in their body. During my sessions with the practitioner, who has a gifted and nurturing touch, she would often work on what she experienced as some rigidity in my spine, which would have a profound effect on my bowel. After our sessions I would leave discomfort-free and with the distinct impression that a process of rejuvenation in my bowel had been triggered. Some level of nourishment of the tissues of my bowel, which had not been possible for many years, had been facilitated. I was also left with the impression that some part of my being had been fundamentally changed as a result of the treatment, the work seeming to address some aspect of my unconscious.

Several times after these treatment sessions I would go directly to an evening at the personal development course. On a couple of occasions I had an experience of myself during the seminar that was quite uncharacteristic and delightfully refreshing. At times during the seminar there would be an opportunity to share with the assembled group an insight or experience that you had had as a result of applying the principles in your everyday life. At these times, despite wanting to stand up and share, I would have to hoist myself out of my chair using my raw willpower to overcome my natural anxiety at exposing my innermost thoughts and feelings in public. Having successfully plucked up the courage to do this, I would sit down usually feeling relieved and pleased that I had been able to overcome my fear and could then be more truly present in the room. However, after the Ortho Bionomy sessions I found myself able to get up and share my thoughts and feelings almost effortlessly, in a way that felt delightfully freeing and did not seem to engage the usual huff and puff and anxiety. Although fragile, a new part of myself seemed to have been engaged, allowing me to come forward into relationship with others in a totally different way.

As a result of these various holistic approaches to healing my bodymind, I have fully regained my physical health and have a renewed sense of vitality and zest for life. A newfound energy and enthusiasm for my work and interactions with people, something that had been missing at some level for several years prior to my illness, is again present in my life. The emotional pain I had been harbouring before getting sick had contributed to a degree of professional burnout and to often feeling drained by my clients. What has been a wonderful and unexpected outcome of my illness has been a far more satisfying experience of my work as a doctor. In becoming less judgemental of my patients, and their inability to take the necessary steps to heal themselves, as I saw it, I have become more receptive to the richness of human interaction that can take place in a consultation. As I have been able to express myself more fully in my work, not feeling bound by some rigid notion of how a doctor should behave, I sense that my ability to serve my patients has improved. Certainly, by being more able to be with my own pain, I have been more able to be with the pain of my patients. This in itself has been a great blessing!

Untying my 'psychic knot'

As much of the focus of my own healing has been directed at the mental and emotional levels of my being, it seems appropriate to say a little about how I understand this complex process. One way of describing what I have been working with over the past four years is to call it a 'psychic knot'. The knot has many different threads caught up in it in a tight jumble. In order to unravel this knot, there first had to be some easing of the tension on the two ends of the string. At a personal level, I needed to create some space in my life, whereby my usual work-a-day pressures were reduced enough to allow examination of this knot. Once this had been achieved it then became possible to gently pull apart the loose ends of the entangled mass. As with most knot untying, I did not have a clear sense of where to begin; it all seemed very confusing. Gradually, however, with patience and determination, I started to get a sense of which threads to pull on. The limiting attitudes and belief systems that had contributed to my disease started to become more obvious and less hidden. In my case there were several different threads that needed to be loosened before the knot could be disentangled, and this process had its own pace and time. The disentangling of the knot required that I get help from other people as there was no way I would have figured it out without the benefit of the wisdom and compassion of a significant number of people.

'The limiting attitudes and belief systems that had contributed to my disease started to become less hidden'

Undoubtedly, my training in Western medicine, yoga and Ayurveda has contributed to how I understand the process of becoming ill with a serious disease and how I've gone about my recovery. The names given to my illness in Western medicine include amoebic ulceration of the large bowel, non-specific colitis and inflammatory bowel disease. Interestingly, in Ayurveda all of these conditions fall under the diagnosis called *grahani* – a complex imbalance of the basic energies of the bodymind which is caused by inappropriate diet and lifestyle as well as emotional and attitudinal factors. The professor of Traditional Chinese Medicine felt that my symptoms were the result of a low intestinal *qi* or life force, which is multifactorial in origin and similar to the Ayurvedic view of why I got sick.

In simple terms, I know that I put a lot of stress into my bowel, something that I have been doing for a long time. My father also suffered from a serious bowel complaint in midlife, which was never properly diagnosed. I now relate to my bowel as the weak link in my body and a sensitive messenger to me of when I am not being true to the deepest part of myself. Whereas prior to my recovery I would internalise my pain and go into a place of anguish, it now became more possible to reach out to others for support and to find ways within myself to move out of these states more quickly.

Ayurveda and yoga acknowledge the central role of the mind in the causation of illness. Mind, in this instance, refers to both its conscious and unconscious elements. Both sciences accept that the body is innately wise and therefore considerable attention is given to listening to the body and the cues, both subtle and gross, that it gives us. These cues can be used to help us live in accordance with our basic nature and can protect us from ill health. In my case a layer of shame contributed to some level of disconnection between my body and my mind. Driven by an army of self-imposed 'shoulds', I had overridden my visceral responses to predicaments I had found myself in. By not acknowledging these bodily reactions, I had energetically weakened the state of the tissues of my bowel, thereby making them more prone to inflammation and ultimately infection.

I can now say that it was my destiny to get sick and to have had an enormous amount of experience, which I would not have otherwise had, as a result of my illness. Given the genes I have inherited from my parents and the accumulated experiences I have had since conception, an illness such as I had was always going to be likely. Just as an acorn thrown into a field will always become an oak tree, all things being equal, so it was only a matter of time before illness would come my way. From the perspective of Ayurveda the fact of my illness was simply a manifestation of how I was out of balance with my essential nature – a product of a life lived with some level of disharmony in regard to the forces of the natural world. To some this may sound overly fatalistic, but as this illness has been a vehicle for profound personal growth and a catalyst for self-acceptance, it has become easier for me to accept the pain and loss that has also come with this learning. I shall finish this brief account of my struggle with ill health with a haiku by the Japanese poet Basho, whose words so beautifully acknowledge life's paradoxes.

My house burnt down
Now I have
A better view
Of the other side.

Conclusion

In reviewing the collective experience of the individuals interviewed for this book a number of clear and unmistakeable themes emerge – themes that I believe will have an important bearing in the twenty-first century as we seek to more fully understand the nature of the healing process. I would now like to recapitulate what I see as the defining features of how these people were able to so positively influence the outcome of the illnesses they have been faced with.

Firstly, they have all stepped forward and been willing to get involved in their own healing. This basic act of taking responsibility for their own health has been fundamental to the process of restoring wellbeing. Rather than leaving their health solely in the hands of health care practitioners, they were able in varied ways to facilitate their healing from serious disease and work in conjunction with their health care practitioners. As a group they displayed a remarkable level of openness to previously untried therapies and treatment approaches. They also showed great persistence in the face of initial 'failures' in pursuing greater health and wellbeing.

Necessarily, each of their paths to recovery has been unique. How they have gone about the process of restoring their health has been very individual. At different times in their healing journeys different approaches have been necessary. Rather than trying to follow a recipe for how to cure a disease from one of the many New Age manuals on offer, they have utilised their natural strengths and gifts to best facilitate their journey towards wellness. Some of the qualities they have brought to bear in the recoveries include pragmatism, intuition, creativity, gritty determination, discriminating intellect and above all courage.

It is also apparent that all of the individuals have taken a holistic approach to their own healing; an approach that recognises the interrelatedness of the different aspects of human experience and that is inclusive of the physical, emotional, mental and spiritual domains of what it is to be a human being. In this view, untoward physical symptoms such as pain or fatigue are seen as signs that there is imbalance in the bodymind; not as things to be got rid of. This movement towards embracing all the different aspects of human experience, including the inevitability of one's own death, rather than disowning those experiences that are difficult or unpleasant in some way, seems to be crucial to their 'successful' outcomes – success, whatever the physical healing that has been achieved, being essentially a subjective experience.

For many of the individuals interviewed the experience of illness has taken them way out of their comfort zones. All of them have had to confront deeply held fears and deal with situations they would not have encountered had they had not been seriously ill. Thus they were given opportunities for learning; opportunities that saw them developing new skills in their day-to-day life, including how to meditate, how to rest, how to breathe more effectively, how to listen to one's body, how to find support, how to nourish oneself through one's diet, how to say 'no', how to express one's feelings and how to acknowledge and get one's needs met in different situations.

Inherent in their journeys towards better health and greater wellbeing has been their ability to take a positive attitude towards their illness. This has meant that, despite the physical and mental suffering that has come with being sick, they have remained open to the experience. They have been able to see that perhaps there have been some important, if hard-won, lessons for them to learn in this lifetime through being sick – even if the nature of those lessons did not become apparent until a considerably later period in their lives.

It is in this context that many of those interviewed have asserted or at least intimated that they saw illness as a gift; a gift in the sense that illness can be a great, if demanding, teacher and a profound vehicle for self-knowledge. This radical shift in perspective has permitted them to move forward into illness as an important life experience, rather than seeing it as a curse or as the result of some negative action committed in the past. This movement forward into the experience of illness allowed for further psychological and emotional growth; growth perhaps not otherwise available to those people.

The lessons learnt by the eight people generous enough to share their stories have much to offer the general public. For people battling serious illness there are some important messages about how best to facilitate the process of self-healing. The medical profession would also do well to take heed of the words of the experiencer of disease, who has for so long been excluded from the health debate.

In the broader social context, we as a community could benefit from embracing illness as a gift and as a valued realm of human experience, despite its difficult nature. An attitude such as this enables healing at the level of the individual as well as of our social institutions, and paves the way to the wholeness that many so desperately seek.

I am struck by the correlations between what these eight individuals have to say about healing and some of the basic tenets of Ayurveda and yoga. As both these traditions draw from wisdom gained from the direct experience of human beings over thousands of years, perhaps it should be no surprise that these correlations emerge.

A uniting theme of indigenous systems of healing is the basic holistic approach they take to understanding human health and disease. In this approach the human being is seen as a body–mind–spirit complex and treatment strategies implicitly or explicitly acknowledge this basic fact. If the Western medical community can stay open to these paradigms of healing, as it is slowly starting to do, and like the people interviewed for this book move beyond its comfort zone, it will undoubtedly be more able to effectively serve the people who seek its help.

Appendix: A story of ancient healing in the modern world

*'There is more in heaven and earth
Horatio, than is dreamt of in your
philosophy.'*
HAMLET, WILLIAM SHAKESPEARE

One of the most pleasing aspects of being involved in the teaching of Ayurveda is that I get to meet some delightful people. Farida Irani, who runs a successful practice as an Ayurvedic aromatherapist/holistic practitioner and regularly brings out Ayurvedic practitioners to give teaching seminars in Australia, is one such person. Farida and her husband Sheriar are both originally from India and lived in Dubai and Iran for fourteen years before migrating to Australia fifteen years ago. They are very passionate about Ayurveda as a healing science.

Farida comes from a Parsi family who live in Bombay and got interested in Ayurveda through her own struggle with ill health. She was involved with yoga and meditation from her teens. Her story is a powerful reminder for me of how much we still don't know about healing, despite the technological advances of recent years. Farida's illness had its origins in a difficult labour she experienced in Dubai in 1982 during which she lost a lot of blood and had to be given a blood transfusion. Despite feeling rundown she returned to full-time work as an accountant, which she found very stressful because it was fraught with office politics. Badly in need of a break and at the insistence of her husband, she later quit her

Appendix: A story of ancient healing in the modern world

job and returned to her native India for a holiday. It was here that she contracted hepatitis A.

The symptoms of hepatitis started several weeks later while she was on a family holiday in Europe, with the onset of fever and nausea. When her urine turned the colour of dark tea a family friend and physician in Italy diagnosed hepatitis and she was advised to return home to Dubai immediately. By the time she arrived at Dubai airport she had turned a mustard yellow colour and was constantly scratching, much to the concern of her fellow passengers on the flight. Her physicians placed her under quarantine in her apartment in Dubai for the next two months.

The Western medical approach to the treatment of hepatitis is based around bed rest and avoiding heavy and fatty foods. Farida also followed the Ayurvedic approach to the treatment of hepatitis and started herself on a special diet of fresh sugar-cane juice and boiled fruit and vegetables. Despite this regimen – her daily rest made possible by her mother's presence in their home and a live-in nanny – Farida's jaundice was still no better six months later. Her liver function tests were markedly raised and in her own words she was 'skin and bone'. Desperate to improve her health Farida again returned to India to get a detailed checkup from one of Bombay's finest physicians. This physician, distressed at how much the hepatitis had damaged her liver, recommended immediate hospitalisation. Farida agreed.

It was at this time that Farida's mother's domestic helper suggested Farida see a healer who was renowned in that part of Bombay in the treatment of jaundice. The man was an illiterate *lalya* (a local indigenous man), who came from a part of Gujarat state where some of India's indigenous people live. He was popular with the local fisher-folk, the Kolis, who live in coastal villages close to the heart of downtown Bombay.

The man was duly contacted and agreed to come and do a few day's treatment on Farida. She refused to ingest anything, bearing in mind that he was not a qualified Ayurvedic physician, and was pleased to discover that his treatments did not involve taking herbs. Apparently, his guru had given him what is called an *ilm*, or mystical gift, of being able to heal jaundice, on condition that he never take money in his hands for his services. Being poor, he would however accept money if it was offered to him, by opening his pocket and allowing the recipient of his treatment to put money in it. Treatments involved the application of some lime-chalk to Farida's arms and legs. The healer, after seeking her permission, moistened the chalk in water and applied it like soap to the skin of her arms, from the elbows down, and to her legs from the knees down. Farida then watched in amazement as the white chalk turned more and more yellow with each pass of the chalk over her skin. She realised that he was draining the excess bile products from her body thus, using the chalk to detoxify her system. Throughout the procedure the healer was also chanting under his breath, and Farida could feel an energy passing through her.

Each session would last around fifteen minutes and she was advised to drink plenty of fresh coconut water and eat only fruit and vegetables. After three consecutive days of treatment, during which the same procedure was followed, the healer asked her to rest for a week then go to the hospital for a repeat test of her liver function. After the third day of her treatment Farida's urine started to get lighter in colour and the repeat liver function test one week later, as with all subsequent liver function tests, was normal. This man had cured her hepatitis, for which Farida has been profoundly grateful ever since. She subsequently rebuilt herself with her regular yoga practice and meditation, things she had let go due to her busy career.

Farida's story is significant as it highlights the importance of honouring the healing traditions of the earth's indigenous people, many of which are being lost in our current age so infatuated with technology and with all that is new. The treasure trove that is contained within the oral traditions of these cultures around the world, including that of Australia's indigenous people, has only received scant attention from modern medical researchers – a regrettable situation and one that is a disservice to humanity as a whole.

Glossary

Acupuncture and Traditional Chinese Medicine: An ancient system of medicine for balancing the flow of vital energy or *chi* (or *qi*) in the body. It is used to improve functioning of the body's internal organs and enhance immunity. Treatments may involve insertion of needles into acupuncture points, dietary and lifestyle advice as well as the prescription of Chinese herbs.

Alexander technique: A method of re-educating the bodymind to improve posture and co-ordination. It was developed by an Australian actor, Frederick Alexander.

Anthroposophical medicine: An approach to healing based on the ideas of Rudolph Steiner, an Austrian visionary and philosopher who wrote in the early part of the twentieth century.

Artha: The material resources that enable one to follow one's *dharma*.

Asanas: Body postures and stretches used in yoga to stimulate the flow of the body's vital energy or *prana*.

Ayurveda: The traditional system of medicine practised in India over the past 5,000 years. It utilises food, herbs, music, colour and aromas as well as yoga postures and meditation to restore balance to the bodymind. Based on the three *doshas* or bodymind principles (*vata*, *pitta* and *kapha*), it seeks to harmonise body, mind and spirit. It is a sister science of yoga.

Bioenergetics: A system of exercises to help individuals become more aware of where they store tension in their bodies and how to relieve such tension. In this way, problems of the mind can be healed through the language of the body.

Bodymind: A word used in complementary medical circles that acknowledges the innate connection between the mind and the body. The human being is seen as a whole rather than the sum of its collective parts. The body, as well as the mind, is seen as intelligent. The term 'bodymind' more accurately reflects an energetic understanding of the human being, as described in Traditional Chinese Medicine and Ayurveda.

Bodywork: An umbrella term used to describe various forms of massage that work on muscles, fascia, joints and soft tissue to restore energy flow and vitality.

Buteyko breathing method: A breathing practice developed by a Russian doctor to assist individuals to breathe more effectively. The method is popular in the treatment of asthma.

Chiropractic medicine: A system of health care that uses spinal and joint manipulation to improve functioning of the nervous system, thereby stimulating the body's natural defences. It originated in the United States in the nineteenth century.

Dharma: At the level of the individual, this refers to that path through life that allows a person to achieve their full potential and fulfil their own unique destiny.

EMDR (Eye Movement Desentisation and Reprocessing): A technique used by psychotherapists to reduce the psychic impact of disturbing images such as flashbacks in people with post-traumatic stress disorder.

Feldenkrais: An approach to enhancing mental and bodily coordination that uses movement and awareness of posture. The founder is an Israeli engineer.

Homeopathy: A system of medicine first propounded by Samuel Hahnemann in Germany in the early nineteenth century. It seeks to manipulate a person's vital force using infinitesimal doses of various substances.

Iridology: A discipline that uses the iris to diagnose constitutional type and to identify inherent structural weaknesses in the body and tissue dysfunction.

Kama: The enjoyment of mundane pleasures such as eating good food, listening to a beautiful piece of music and enjoying one's children.

Kinesiology: A therapeutic approach that uses muscle testing to identify structural, chemical and mental imbalance. Wellbeing is then restored using gentle manipulation, exercise and diet.

Macrobiotics: A way of living and eating that recognises the natural order in all things physical, mental, ecological and spiritual. The macrobiotic approach to food draws from Traditional Chinese Medicine, with foods being classified as either yin (negative, dark, feminine) or yang (positive, bright, masculine).

Meditation: The process whereby the mind is brought into balance in different situations and life circumstances. This may involve specific mental practices where the mind is focused on a specific image, sensation or subtle sound.

Meridians: Line of energy along which the vital energy or *chi* travels, as described in traditional Chinese Medicine.

Moksha: This relates to the spiritual domain of one's life and finding liberation from the misery of the human condition and cycle of death and rebirth.

Naturopathy: A health care system that uses various approaches to enhance healing, including food, herbs, vitamins and minerals as well as massage. Most naturopaths are trained in iris diagnosis.

Ortho Bionomy: A type of bodywork that seeks to restore natural functioning of the body through gentle postural realignment.

Osteopathy: A system of medical practice that originated in the United States in the nineteenth century. It uses gentle manipulation of the musculo-skeletal system to restore blood supply to the organs of the body, thereby allowing healing to take place.

Pathologise: To view physical or mental experiences as expressions of a diseased state.

Pranayama: Breathing practices used in yoga to enhance the flow of energy in the bodymind which are purifying in nature.

Psychoneuroimmunology: An emerging field of study and clinical practice in Western medicine which acknowledges the fundamental connections between the mind, the nervous system, the body's hormones and the immune system.

Qi gong: A self-healing practice from China that uses movement, breathing and meditation to strengthen the body's *qi* or vital energy. It is useful in the promotion of health, fitness and longevity and as an adjunct in the treatment of chronic disease.

Reflexology: A therapeutic method that uses manual pressure to specific areas of the feet to activate natural healing in other parts of the body. It is also known as Zone Therapy.

Reiki: An approach to healing originally from Japan that uses gentle touch to balance the energy of the bodymind and to promote healing.

Shiatsu: A system of massage originally from Japan that works on specific energy channels to restore proper functioning of the organs of the body. It is usually done through clothes.

Somatic psychotherapy: An approach to psychotherapy that recognises the whole body as a map of our unconscious. Attitudes and deep emotions held in the tissues of the body are explored in therapy to bring about a more relaxed and functional approach to living. A somatic psychotherapist is able to assess energy flow through the body and can help one learn how to restore the movement of energy in the body. This can profoundly influence mental and physical wellbeing.

T'ai chi: A system of movements and postures based on an ancient Chinese philosophy designed to encourage the movement of the body's vital force or *chi*. It is useful in the promotion of health, fitness and longevity.

Vedanta: A school of philosophy and spiritual practice from India.

Vedic architecture: A sister science of Ayurveda also known as Vaastu. It is an ancient Indian science that concerns itself with how to create built environments that bring wellbeing and harmony to their users.

Vedic astrology (also called 'Jyotish'): This sister science of Ayurveda is the astrology from which Western astrology branched. It incorporates a holistic view of the mundane, psychological and spiritual aspects of human life.

Vipassana meditation: A Buddhist meditation practice where individuals focus their attention on subtle and gross sensations around the body.

Yoga: A tradition of spiritual practice from India where individuals seek to unite themselves with the godhead. A number of non-exclusive paths cater for individuals of different temperaments. Some of the main paths are: (1) Raja Yoga – involves moral training, physical postures (*asanas*), breathing practices (*pranayama*), meditation and eating wholesome foods. This path has become popular in Western countries in recent times. (2) Hatha Yoga – seeks to purify the body using cleansing practises, physical postures and breathing practices. It is a preliminary path to Raja Yoga. (3) Karma Yoga – the path of selfless service, of which Mahatma Gandhi is an example. (4) Bhakti Yoga – the path of devotion, usually to a specific aspect of the divine, such as a deity or an enlightened teacher. (5) Jnana Yoga – the path of wisdom, generally suited to those with an intellectual disposition. (6) Tantric Yoga – seeks to broaden one's range of mental experiences in the development of consciousness, using rituals, mantras, *pranayama* and meditation.

Yoga therapy: The application of the principles of yoga in the treatment of physical and mental disease. A yoga therapist, as well as being an experienced yoga teacher, usually has also undergone training in another health science such as medicine, nursing, naturopathy, physiotherapy or osteopathy.

Acknowledgements

Many people have contributed to the writing of this book. I would especially like to express my gratitude to:

My literary agent Fiona Inglis for her enthusiasm and belief in me from the very beginning.

Sally Cullen and Frank Formby whose critical feedback and encouragement after reading the first draft of this book were invaluable.

My mother Wendy Matthews who generously offered to transcribe the tape recordings of the interviews and for her support throughout this five-year process.

Joanne Albany for her patience and devoted care of our son during the writing of this book.

Peter Broughton for his meticulous proofreading and warm support.

John Swindells whose challenging comments and sensitive understanding of the essence of this book have been much appreciated.

Adrian House whose wealth of experience in how to communicate more effectively with one's readers helped enormously in the editing of this book.

Barry de Ferranti for his computer nous and encouragement along the way.

Carole Marando, Cheryl Flint, Francoise Masson and Paolo Bassi who read some of the initial drafts of this book and made some very useful suggestions.

Rex Finch, publisher of Finch Publishing, for his strong acknowledgement of the worth of this project and for taking me on as an unknown writer.

Marie-Louise Taylor and Sean Doyle, my editors at Finch Publishing, whose enthusiasm, humour and wise counsel made the editing of this book a most rewarding process.

Julianne Sheedy and Oonagh Kalsy of Finch Publishing, and my publicist Sue-Anna Purcell.

Nanette Backhouse for her fine work with the front cover.

Susan Boyle for the artwork inside the book.

Ian Gawler, for graciously agreeing to write the Foreword and for being such an inspiring role model over the years.

I also want to honour all the individuals who have agreed to share their stories so generously and courageously. Without them *Journeys in Healing* would never have come into being.

Further reading

Vedanta
Balsekar, Ramesh S., *Consciousness Speaks*, Advaita Press, Bombay, 1992.
Sri Nisargadatta Maharaj, *I Am That*, Chetana Press, Redondo Beach, 1973.

Ayurveda
Lad, Vasant, *Ayurveda: The Science of Self-Healing*, Lotus Press, Wisconsin, 1984.
Svoboda, Robert E., *Ayurveda: Life, Health and Longevity*, Penguin Books, London, 1992.
Svoboda, Robert E., *Prakruti: Your Ayurvedic Constitution*, Geocom, Albuquerque, 1989.

Death and dying
Kübler-Ross, Elisabeth, *On Death and Dying*, Tavistock, London, 1970.
Levine, Stephen, *Who Dies?* Doubleday, New York, 1982.

Spiritual life and psychology
Bedi, Ashok, *Path to the Soul*, Samuel Weiser, Maine, 2000.

Meditation
Gawler, Ian, *Peace of Mind*, Hill of Content, Melbourne, 1987.

Mind–body medicine
Cousins, Norman, *Anatomy of an Illness*, Bantam Books, New York, 1979.
Gawler, Ian, *You Can Conquer Cancer*, Hill of Content, Melbourne, 1984.
Goleman, Daniel [editor] *Mindbody Medicine*, Choice, Sydney, 1995.
Martin, Paul, *The Sickening Mind*, Flamingo, London, 1997.

Somatic psychotherapy
Keleman, Stanley, *Emotional Anatomy*, Center Press, Berkeley, 1985.
Keleman, Stanley, *Your Body Speaks its Mind*, Center Press, Berkeley, 1975.
Lowen, Alexander, *Bioenergetics*, Penguin Books, New York, 1975.
Lowen, Alexander, *The Spirituality of the Body*, Macmillan, New York, 1990.

Yoga
Desikachar, T. K. V., *The Heart of Yoga*, Inner Traditions International, Rochester, Vermont, 1995.
Mohan, A. G., *Yoga for Body, Breath and Mind*, Rudra Press, Madras, 1993.
Saraswati, Swami Satyananda, *Asana Pranayama Mudra Bandha*, Bihar School of Yoga, Bihar, 1996.

Other Finch titles of interest

Manhood: *An action plan for changing men's lives* (Third edition)
Steve Biddulph tackles the key areas of a man's life – parenting, love and sexuality, finding meaning in work, and making real friends. He presents new pathways to healing the past and forming true partnerships with women, as well as honouring our own inner needs. ISBN 1876451 203

Stories of Manhood: *Journeys into the hidden hearts of men*
Steve Biddulph presents his selection of the best writings from around the world on the inner lives of men. Powerful, funny, and heart-rending, these stories show that men are infinitely larger than the narrow stereotypes they are given. ISBN 1876451 106

Older Men's Business
Valuing relationships, living with change
Jack Zinn
In this important book, men aged 55 and over talk about adjusting to major life changes, their personal relationships and the challenges they face. ISBN 1876451 335

The Myth of Male Power
Why men are the disposable sex
Dr Warren Farrell presents a significant and well-researched plea against the image of male-as-oppressor, arguing that this misconception has hindered not only men, but women too. ISBN 1876451 300

Dealing with Anger
Self-help solutions for men
Frank Donovan
Focussing on emotional healing and practical change, this book includes case studies from clients of the author's (a psychotherapist) and a program of exercises for the reader.
ISBN 1876451 05X

The Body Snatchers
How the media shapes women
Cyndi Tebbel
From childhood, women are told they can never be too thin or too young. The author exposes the rampant conditioning of women and girls by those pushing starvation imagery, and encourages us to challenge society's preoccupation with an ideal body that is unnatural and (for most) unattainable. ISBN 1876451 076

Blood Ties
The stories of five positive women
Edited by Salli Trathen
This collection of the stories of five Australian HIV-positive women reveals how each woman approached her predicament, and the inner qualities she drew on to persevere. The authors' honest and courageous writing allows us to live with them through their struggles. What emerges is a triumph of the human spirit over adversity. ISBN 1 876451 297

Kids Food Health: *Nutrition and your child's development*
The authors, Dr Patricia McVeagh – a paediatrician – and Eve Reed – a dietitian – present the parents of children from newborns to teenagers with the latest information on the impact of diet on health, growth, allergies, behaviour and physical development.
Kids Food Health 1: *The first year* ISBN 1876451 149
Kids Food Health 2: *From toddler to preschooler* ISBN 1876451 157
Kids Food Health 3: *From school-age to teenage* ISBN 1876451 165

Women Can't Hear What Men Don't Say
Destroying myths, creating love
Dr Warren Farrell provides a remarkable communication program to assist couples in understanding and loving each other more fully. ISBN 1876451 319

Side by Side
How to think differently about your relationship
Jo Lamble and Sue Morris provide helpful strategies to overcome the pressures that lead to break-ups, as well as valuable advice on communication, problem-solving and understanding the stages in new and established relationships. A marvellous book for young people. ISBN 1876451 092

Online and Personal
The reality of Internet relationships
With the boom in Internet dating services and chat rooms, authors Jo Lamble and Sue Morris offer guidelines for Net users to protect themselves, their relationships and their children from the hazards that exist online. ISBN 1876451 173

For further information on these and all of our titles, visit our website: www.finch.com.au

Index

Aboriginal healing 225–26
acupuncture 51, 152–53
advice, reaction to 131
agni 155–57
allergies 137, 142
artha 183
asthma
  contributory factors 134, 136–37, 186–87
  effect of 133–35, 137
  healing process 138–42, 186
  overcome 132, 136
Ayurveda
  aims of 181–84
  bowel disease 235
  diet 113, 213
  principles of 155–58
  role of the mind 236
  teaching 215–17
  tradition of 212–14
  treatment style 216–17

behaviour patterns 185–86, 189–90, 191
belief systems 188–89, 217
body, listening to 176–77
body image, women's 28
bodywork 110–11, 178–79, 211–12
breathing techniques 24, 44, 97, 138, 139, 154, 177
bronchodilators 133, 134, 137
Buteyko breathing 24, 154, 177

cancer, self-healing 9, 207
change, embracing 171–72
childhood health
  Nicki 16–17, 20
  Shankardev 133–35
'child's eyes' 99–100
Chinese medicine 117, 150–51
chronic fatigue syndrome (CFS)
  contributory factors 38–39, 44, 176, 178, 185–86
  effect of 32–35, 36, 189
  healing practices 30, 42–44, 105–7, 110–11, 179
  onset of 30, 104
  others' reaction 109, 162, 179
  symptoms and diagnosis of 30–32, 105
communication skills, teaching 165–66
community, sense of 118–19
consciousness 39–40, 135, 144, 169
consultations 152
Contact Improvisation 125, 126

control, psychological 26, 28–29
counselling 72
Cushing's disease
  contributory factors 88, 186
  diagnosis 84
  effect of 84–86, 93, 95, 164
  healing practices 93–97
  relapse 89
  surgery for 84

Dalai Lama 185
dancing 93–94, 124, 125–28, 155, 171
death 64–65, 66, 73, 170, 190, 205–6
denial 26
depression 36
detoxification 139–40
dharma 181–83
diagnosis, reaction to 69, 148–49, 219–21
diet
  anti-candida 94
  Ayurvedic 113, 213
  vegetarian 18
digestion, process of 156–57

eisteddfod experience 63–64, 197
emotional healing 188
empathy, need for 165–67

fees, medical 165
financial difficulties 26–27, 119, 165, 196

Gawler, Ian 207–8
God, attitude towards 61–62, 77, 90, 93, 100, 164
grieving, stages of 149
grounding 96–97

healing
  approaches to 152–54, 170, 175–78
  four quadrants of 59, 187–92
  holistic 221–22
  learning from 60
  process of 25, 46, 59, 78–79, 101–2, 115–16, 129–30, 143–44, 194
  understanding 169–70
heart–lung damage
  Buteyko breathing 154
  emotional effect 16–17
  heart–lung transplant program 17–18, 25–26

  symptoms 15–16
  treatment 17–19, 25
hepatitis A treatment 241–42
HIV virus
  contributory factors 72–73
  early testing for 68–69
  effects of 67, 70, 79–80
  healing practices 70–71, 76–78, 169–70
  other illnesses and 71, 74
  others' reaction to 69–70, 74, 162
  positive results from 72
holidays 27
holistic medical practice 216–17
hospitalisation 15, 17, 22, 24, 166
human contact, need for 166
humour, sense of 23, 64, 190, 197–98

illness
  contributory factors to 98, 194, 218–19
  facing 27–29, 66, 80–82, 102–3, 117, 134, 144–45
  as a gift 39–40, 62–63, 65–66
  learning from 60, 82, 100–101, 114–15, 141–43, 144, 175, 178–80
  negative aspects of 40–41, 74–75, 93, 108–9, 196
  positive aspects of 21–23, 41–42, 75–76, 92, 110, 125, 138, 166–67, 172–73, 190–91, 195–99
  psychological factors 185–87
  reasons for 219–21
  role of the mind 236
  self-blame for 161–62, 175
  speaking about 56–57, 162, 179–80, 188
  uncertainty of 86
  unrelated to disease 36
immune system function 158
inner resources 130, 168–71, 173–74
integration, process of 54–57
Irani, Farida 240–42
iridology 209
isolation, social 40–41, 78, 162–63, 164, 179, 227–28

Joshua's story 183
journal keeping 44, 52, 95

Kahuna massage 211
kama 183
King, Petrea 41–42

250 Journeys in Healing

koshas 193
Kriya yoga 139–40

laughter 197–98
life
  in charge of 61
  getting on with 99–100, 123
lifestyle changes 33–35, 37–38,
    171–72, 189, 191–92, 198–99
love 60–61, 62

marijuana 53, 135
massage
  Ayurvedic 182
  Chinese 226–27
  Cushing's disease 94–95, 96, 98
  Kahuna form 211
  self-massage 96
  Zen shiatsu 128–29
Matthews, Dr Shaun
  attends cancer retreat 207–8
  Ayurvedic training 213–16
  effect of own illness 166–67
  healing process 221–36
  ill health of 218–34
  medical training 202–17
  sets up holistic medical centre 209
  studies somatic psychology 210–12
  studies yoga 215
  Tibetan experience 204–6
meditation
  asthma 138
  CFS 44, 45, 106
  HIV virus 76
  psychotic episodes 52, 53, 57–58,
    153–54, 170, 177–78
mental healing 188–90
mental health 157
mind, role in illness 236
mindfulness 115, 191
moksha 183–84
moment, living in the 43, 77, 82,
    115, 191
myalgic encephalomyelitis (ME) *see*
  chronic fatigue syndrome (CFS)

negativity 28, 102–3

opening up 55–57
Ortho Bionomy 233, 234

panic attacks 107
parents
  concern of 49
  grief of 122–23
  relationship with 54
perfectionism 87–88, 89, 113, 172,
    189, 197
personal development course 230–34
physical healing 187–88
post-traumatic stress disorder 104,
    178

proactive behaviour 26, 27–29,
    149–59, 168–71
'psychic knot,' untying 234–36
psychoneuroimmunology 158–59
psychotherapy 210–11, 222–23
psychotic episodes
  contributory factors 47–50, 53
  eating habits 52–53
  healing practices 51–52, 54–59
  loss of reality 48–49, 50, 51
  meditation 53, 57–58, 153–54,
    170, 177–78
  others' reaction to 179
  positive aspects of 196–97

quadriplegia
  acceptance of 170–71
  cause of 120
  dancing 124, 125–28, 155, 171
  emotional aspects of 121–23, 164
  physical extent of 121

radiotherapy 84–85
rapid eye movement desensitisation
    106
reading 62
reality, losing touch with 48
'rebirth' 50, 56, 116
recovery, belief in 130–31
rejection and HIV virus 74–75
relapse, fear of 36–37
relationships
  effect on illness 88, 89–91, 186,
    222–23
  with parents 54, 222, 230, 232
  stress on 162–63
relaxation process 113–14

saltwater cleansing 140
self, sense of 45–46, 108–9, 112, 116,
    160–61, 197, 199, 220
self-destruction 73, 100
self-doubt 163–65
self-examination 172–73
self-healing 141–43, 153–55,
    168–71, 173–74
self-massage 96, 98
self-regulation 142–43, 176
self-responsibility 101–3, 112–13,
    149–51
sexual identity 164, 189
smoking 50, 62–63
social situations 35, 38, 40, 112,
    133–35, 162–63, 179, 223
somatic psychotherapy 96–97, 106,
    107–8, 154, 171–72, 176, 190,
    210–11
spiritual healing 190–92, 224–25
strength, sources of 23–24, 45–46,
    77–78, 98, 114, 129, 141, 168–71
support
  accepting 118, 180

by family 57–58, 123, 162–63
by friends 16–17, 19, 20, 124,
    162–63, 180
lack of 33, 134
positive 102–3
professional 28
spiritual 58
support groups
  CFS 114, 153
  community networks 118–19
  Cushing's disease 91–92
  dislike for 35
  HIV virus 75
swimmers' muscle 121

t'ai chi 51
thalidomide
  availability of 14
  compensation 26–27
  organ damage from 15
  see also heart-lung damage
Tibetan medicine 205–6
touch 93
Traditional Chinese Medicine 117,
    150–51
trust 45–46

uncertainty 163–65

values, of society 144
Vedanta 45, 178
Vedic astrology 215
Vipassana meditation 52, 53, 76,
    177–78
visualisation 86–87

weakness, perception of 35–36, 137,
    161
wellness, definition of 37
Western medical system 81
wheelchair
  adjusting to 122–23
  freedom from 128
  reaction to 164, 171
willpower 173–74

yoga
  asthma 135–36, 138–43, 154
  breathing techniques 138, 139,
    177
  CFS 34, 44
  Cushing's disease 95–96
  Desikachar style 112–13
  Kriya 139–40
  principles of 192–94
  quadriplegia 126
  relaxing approach to 172, 176
  author's experience of 214–15

Zen shiatsu massage 128–29